SHADOW SUMMIT

ONE MAN, HIS DIAGNOSIS, AND
THE ROAD TO A VIBRANT LIFE

A MEMOIR BY
JON CHANDONNET

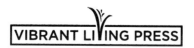
VIBRANT LIVING PRESS

Text and Layout Design: Worthy Marketing Group
Cover Design: Worthy Marketing Group

LCCN: 2013911179

ISBN 978-0-615-83656-0

Printed in the United States of America

TABLE OF CONTENTS

A note to the reader:

My relationship with multiple sclerosis began with denial: running marathons, climbing mountains, and working eighty-hour weeks. Living with MS, I have experienced sorrows and, more importantly, great joys, like having a child and deepening my connection with my wife, my family, my friends, and myself. MS re-created who I am and what I want.

I do not have a medical degree or training. Though I share insights about my healing, this book is not a roadmap to recovery. I just want to tell my story about coming to terms with a disease that many people consider a death sentence. MS changed my life in ways I could have never imagined and in ways that have made my life better. I hope my story offers inspiration and hope.

Jon Chandonnet

Santa Monica, California

All truths are easy to understand once they are discovered;
the point is to discover them.

- Galileo

PART I
OPENING

1

THE BEGINNING

I stood above the free throw line and helplessly watched the ball sail toward my opponent. He caught it and made a strong move to the basket. I threw my body in front of him, but my defense wasn't pretty.

My left leg, usually quick to react, was rooted to the floor like a tree stump. My calf and quad muscles locked, ignoring the command to act. My left arm was equally unresponsive. I wanted to put my hand in front of the ball and follow my opponent, but no matter how much I tried, I couldn't get my arm where it needed to be. It lacked its usual strength and agility. It flailed in front of me rather than extending deftly above my head to reach for the ball. When I sparred in Tae Kwan Do, I could put my foot or fist in my opponent's chest before he knew what hit him. Now I was the one taken by surprise.

I was in the midst of one of those nightmares where I stood paralyzed, unable to flee an attacker, except I was wide-awake in the middle of a basketball game. It took all my strength and focus to lunge with my right leg and drag my left into my opponent's path. My mind knew where my left arm and leg needed to be, but my body wasn't getting the message. I knew my jerky, awkward movements caught the attention of my teammates, and I became self-conscious.

Not surprisingly, the other team scored.

I turned and hurried down the court; my body jack-knifed, herky-jerky as I ran. When I finally made it to the other end of the floor, I tried to get into the offensive flow. I set a pick, but my left side wasn't cooperating. I thought I might have pulled a muscle, but this feeling—whatever it was—was different than anything I'd ever felt before, and I was starting to freak out. I raised my right arm, the good one, and called for a substitute. I told everyone, including myself, I had pulled a muscle. I wanted to save face and didn't want to let my teammates down.

I walked to the bench and took a seat. When I caught my breath, I sat on the floor and massaged my left leg and vigorously shook my left arm to see if I could get a response. I knew it was just an intramural game and not the NBA finals, so I told my teammates I was out for the rest of the half. At halftime I took Matt, the team captain and my best buddy, aside and tried to explain.

"Dude, I think I pulled a muscle on my left side. It's my leg or back; I'm not sure. I don't think I should play the second half."

"No problem, the team will cover for you."

I was thankful he was so cool and sat on the bench for the rest of the game, rooting our team to victory. When it was over, I went home and stretched my leg again, but it didn't help. Though I had a limp, I was able to ride my bike to MIT every day to attend class and work on my thesis. I also continued my twice-weekly Tae Kwan Do workouts as well, but only worked out on the heavy bag because my left leg and arm didn't have the responsiveness needed to land accurate punches and kicks.

Over a week and a half had passed since the night on the basketball court, and it seemed strange there was still lack of strength and responsiveness on my left side. Though I couldn't attend formal Tae Kwan Do class, my symptoms didn't prevent me from working out or going to school, so I looked past them. I was a young, naïve guy who thought I was invincible. I refused to let a pulled muscle slow me down.

After another week, my arm and leg regained some responsiveness but hadn't returned to normal, so I called the student health center, got the name of an internist, Dr. Heller, and scheduled an appointment. I had waited more than two weeks to make the appointment because I convinced myself I was too busy; and I didn't want to be inconvenienced if the result meant I'd have to endure a special regimen for treatment.

The previous year, I visited the medical center to receive treatment for optic neuritis, a condition where the myelin sheath surrounding my right eye's optic nerve unraveled. I realized something was wrong while I was studying for my first-semester statistics final. I couldn't focus—it was like looking through a pane of cracked glass as I read; words were jumbled and blurry. I worried my vision problems might be something major, but rather than engage my fear and anxiety, I ignored the symptoms.

I studied even more to compensate for the time I was losing because of my damaged eyesight. I hoped it would pass. I was too young to have a major health problem. I didn't tell my statistics professor because I didn't want him to think I wanted an excuse to get out of the exam. I was the last person to turn in my test, but I finished.

After finals, I returned home to Philadelphia to celebrate Christmas and New Year's. I had a family friend, a prominent ophthalmologist in the area, diagnose me. The treatment was a week of daily, hour-long, intravenous steroid infusions that I took during my first week back at school during winter break at MIT—involving six weeks of independent study. Fortunately, my eyesight returned to normal before my spring-semester classes began, and I forgot about my troubles. I hoped we would be able to treat my arm and leg problems just as easily, and that those, too, would just disappear.

I told Dr. Heller about the night on the basketball court and my history with optic neuritis. He tested my reflexes and asked for more details about my health history: mono at sixteen and a bout with phantom fatigue at nineteen. He tested my balance, strength, and coordination, and seeing I was in good shape, couldn't determine anything wrong. He recommended I see Dr. Book, a neurologist on staff, just to be sure. Now we were getting somewhere. I hoped the specialist would put this phantom muscle pull to rest.

Dr. Book looked me over thoroughly and performed the same balance, coordination, and strength exercises that Dr. Heller had done. Although the stiffness in my leg and the lack of responsiveness had dissipated somewhat, Dr. Book recommended an MRI of my brain to rule out a neurological issue. The first available appointment was in three weeks, so I took it, wanting to get back to my old life. I was on track to graduate from MIT, and I refused to let anything stop me.

♦

I wasn't thrilled to climb into the MRI tube, but I drifted off to sleep after the technician talked me through the procedure. After it was over, I hopped off the table and dressed for the subway ride back to campus, anxious to get back to classes. On my way out, the technician told me the results of my MRI would be ready in about two weeks. I didn't talk to anyone, family or friends, about my health or about the brain scan. I had always been a minimalist and didn't see the point. Less was more was my thinking at the time, though it would cost me later. I passed the time waiting for the MRI results with thesis interviews, Tae Kwan Do, and school. I tried not to brood over what my life might look like after the results. Instead, I distracted myself with a job search.

I hadn't looked for a job before then because Matt and I had been talking about starting a company based on the independent study project we were doing to create a virtual tour of the MIT campus. We had created a rough business plan and even agreed on a name, Virtual View. I was committed to the idea but knew we had a long way to go to get the business up and running. The truth is I was thinking about a different future. After all that interaction with the medical community, I knew it was naïve to consider only one career option.

I received a lead on a job during a recent conversation with my dad. He and my mom had been out to dinner with friends while vacationing in Florida and had met another couple, Mike and Stewart Moore. Their son, Stuart, was co-CEO of a fast growing software development company, Sapient Corporation, headquartered in Cambridge at the edge of the MIT campus. My dad spoke with Mike about my accomplishments and aspirations. Mike recommended that I give his son a call to talk about career opportunities—Sapient was looking for bright, motivated young people.

I set up a time to see Stuart. As I walked across campus to Sapient's offices, I still had a slight limp that I assumed was indiscernible because none of my classmates had asked about it. As long as I could do what I wanted and needed, the MRI results seemed like an after-thought. My body seemed to be taking care of the damage, granted it was at a slower pace than I would have liked.

Sapient's office impressed me immediately. I suspected the choice offices at One Memorial Drive must have commanding views of the Charles River, a clear indicator of the company's success. Dressed in my best suit and tie, I took the elevator to the fifth floor and when the door opened, I saw the Charles River through the glass walls.

I walked up to the receptionist and asked for Stuart Moore. I had never met with such an esteemed member of the corporate community and felt more than a little self-conscious, but I wore my game face and took a seat. Everyone who walked past was dressed in the same professional attire and had a similar sense of urgency and focus. While it was a more formal environment than the campus of MIT, it was equally as intense, and I felt like I was supposed to be there.

Stuart walked out of his office and invited me into the conference room, where the afternoon sun reflected brilliantly off the river. Stuart was a young guy, in his early forties, with a kind face and relaxed manner. While I knew I hadn't yet been accepted as a member of his club, in his presence I felt like I had been given access to the kingdom.

Stuart and I spoke for the next twenty minutes about my background and professional aspirations, and he gave me an overview of the company: Sapient had been in business for six years, had grown nearly 100% each of those years and had built a strong international reputation for building trust and gaining client confidence for the custom software applications it developed. I was impressed by the company's unique culture and signature values. Sapient sounded like a great place to begin my career.

After the interview, Stuart invited me to speak with a hiring coordinator who asked if I was interested in returning two days later to participate in a round of interviews. I walked out of the office and into the elevator. My mind was spinning.

The MRI results were ready. I walked through campus to the medial center, experiencing a slight limp as I approached Dr. Heller's office. It seemed strange that he would give me the results since Dr. Book ordered the test. I hoped this didn't mean there was a problem. I wanted to put all of this behind me.

"How's the thesis going?" Dr. Heller began.

"Good. I finish the interviews today and have already started to write about the implications of the World Wide Web for local planning agencies."

"Great," he said. Then he picked up a folder, "I have the results of your MRI."

He stood there and stared. I nodded, waiting for him to continue.

"Jon, the MRI shows you have multiple sclerosis."

I was only twenty-seven. I paused and looked down to consider those two words. *Multiple sclerosis.* It felt like the first time I'd ever heard them. I wished it was the last time. I learned later that 400,000

Americans, roughly one out of every one thousand, has MS. I was a new member of this group, but it wasn't one I was ready to join.

"MS. Really?" I exhaled like someone had landed a roundhouse kick to my gut.

The doctor nodded. "The MRI shows you have a couple of lesions on your brain."

Questions flooded my mind. Multiple sclerosis. What was it? What did it mean? What should I do? As much as I wanted to know the answers, I was in shock and short on time. The last thing I wanted to do was sit there and hear more about a disease that might divert my focus and slow me down. I had to complete my thesis interviews. I hoped the doctor would give me the abridged version so I could be on my way.

"Multiple sclerosis is a condition where the immune system attacks the nervous system, so it's an autoimmune disease. The attacked areas on the nerves are left with scar tissue, lesions, where myelin, the protective covering around the nerve, wears away."

"Myelin?" I asked, feeling dislocated by my new reality.

"Myelin is insulation around the nerve that allows signals from the brain to travel uninterrupted to their destination. When the myelin deteriorates, signals that travel along the nerves and hit a de-myelinated area are disrupted and don't reach their intended destination."

I felt nauseous, afraid the doctor would say more. I wanted him to stop so I could get on with my day—thesis interviews, Tae Kwan Do practice, and homework.

"What can I do to treat it?"

"I'm not sure of treatment options, so you need to see Dr. Book."

I put on my backpack and turned to thank the doctor for his time. As I stood and stared into space, he offered some advice: "Don't let the diagnosis rule your life, Jon. Science is moving fast to discover new treatment options all the time."

I nodded, unsure. Before I left, he looked me in the eye one last time and offered the best protocol to follow. "Now go out and live a great life."

♦

I walked to the computer lab in a daze and ran into Matt before I entered.

"Hey, how ya doin'?" he said when he saw me.

I blurted out my news.

"I just found out I have multiple sclerosis."

A look of anguish flashed across his face. "Jon . . . I'm so sorry."

Matt stood to hear more, but I didn't offer anything, and he didn't press. I was still in shock and could not share anything more. The news was too new and too big for me to have a rational discussion about how I felt, much less about what I needed. Several hours later, I left the lab, walked downstairs to get my bike for my ride home and saw my buddy, Terry. We were pretty close, and I thought about whether or not I should tell him. The news was still fresh enough that I hadn't decided *not* to tell anyone just yet.

"Do you have a minute? I have something to tell you," I said.

"Sure."

"I was just diagnosed with multiple sclerosis."

When I said MS, Terry looked like I punched him in the gut.

"Wow, man, I'm so sorry. Matt told me. Are you okay, do you need anything?"

I needed to ignore his question. I needed for someone to tell me the bad dream that had started on the basketball court would end today. Terry gave me a great opportunity to discuss how I felt, but I ignored it. I needed to get to the car rental agency to drive to my afternoon thesis appointments. I needed to get on with my day—and with my life, so we said our good-byes.

As I drove to my meetings, the doctor's advice passed through my mind: *Go out and live a great life*. I thought about what I knew about the disease: not much. I had a family friend with Multiple Sclerosis who lived a life of decreased mobility and was confined to a wheelchair twenty years after the diagnosis. That didn't fit my plans. I would soon graduate with a master's degree in City and Regional Planning from MIT, and then possibly work for our start-up or Sapient Corporation. I imagined a bright future as a leader in the exploding Internet economy, and MS was nowhere in the picture.

Then I remembered I had another family friend who, after an initial MS attack, never experienced any other symptoms. I still had contact with her family and know that after fifteen years, she continued to live symptom free. That was the future I wanted. Maybe a life free from MS was possible for me too?

When I got home after the interviews and Tae Kwan Do, I called my parents.

"Dad, there's something I need to tell you."

"Is everything okay?" Even over the phone, the concern in my dad's voice was clear. It was hard talking to him, especially about something like MS. My relationship with my dad had always been practical, leaving little room for emotions.

I steadied my voice. "I have some bad news about the MRI. The doctor said I had a couple of lesions on my brain that are consistent with multiple sclerosis."

My mom jumped on the second line and I repeated what I told my dad. The line fell silent.

I told them that I didn't know much at this point about the next steps for treatment. I repeated the information I had just learned from Dr. Heller, the same rational way I had been trained, as a child, to deal with difficult emotional circumstances.

"MS is de-myelination of the protective covering around the nerves in my brain, like insulation on a pipe."

Then I explained that since myelin was protective covering around the nerves, de-myelination is the wearing away of the insulation. It's like the padding wearing away on a pipe resulting in a faulty conductor. During an MS attack, signals traveling along the nervous system hit a patch of de-myelinated nerve and don't reach their destination.

There was an extended silence before my dad asked the next logical question. "What's the course of treatment?"

"I don't know. I scheduled an appointment with Dr. Book, my neurologist, on Friday." There was another pause on the line. My dad broke the silence. "We're coming this weekend for a visit. We'll stay at your Aunt Sue's in Marblehead."

My dad's only sister had dealt with family emergencies on short notice before. As a child, my mother had been hospitalized twice after bi-polar episodes when we lived in Vermont. Aunt Sue made the three-hour drive from Marblehead to take care of us.

"It'll be great to see you," I said, relieved.

"How are you feeling otherwise?" my mom asked as her voice cracked.

I could tell she was upset. I told her I'd stopped at my favorite Mexican place for dinner. I assumed this would help settle her motherly concern—let her know I was eating, taking care of myself. I told them the fine motor control in my hand and leg had improved since the basketball game because I just had a great Tae Kwon Do workout.

After I hung up, I called my brother, Pete, who lived in Boulder, Colorado. He is two years older and was always concerned about my welfare, even when we were kids.

I didn't know how to say it so I got right to the point.

"I have some bad news."

"What's up?"

"I've been diagnosed with multiple sclerosis."

I immediately asked if he knew what MS was.

"I've heard of it, but I'm not sure what it is."

I repeated what I told my parents, slowly becoming a student of my own disease.

"How are you feeling?" he asked.

I wasn't ready to open up, not to anyone—especially myself, but I was eager to let him know I was okay. I told him I completed my thesis interviews, rode my bike to school, and attended Tae Kwan Do. Repetition and order were holding my world together. Emotions, I believed, would only destroy it.

"Is there anything I can do for you?"

"No, Mom and Dad are coming up this weekend, and I'm building a network of doctors, but thanks. I need to go do some homework. I'll call this weekend."

"All right, Jon. Call if you need anything."

Friday morning I went to my appointment with Dr. Book. I sat in his office to hear more about the diagnosis. He reiterated that it was an autoimmune disease where the immune system attacks the nervous system. I asked him the only question that really mattered to me at the time "Is there a cure?"

"No, not today, but there's a promising new drug on the market, Betaseron, that shows signs of reducing the occurrence of episodes."

He assured me there were many ongoing studies about the cause and treatment of the disease. Then he explained that there are three different kinds of MS. One is relapsing- remitting, marked by periods of attack then remission in which a person is often able to regain complete motor function. The others are primary- and secondary- progressive, more aggressive types that lead to gradual paralysis in the affected areas.

"Which one do I have?"

"Probably relapsing-remitting, which is marked by attacks and periods of remission where the body is able to recover. The optic neuritis last year was the first attack, and you seem to be fully recovered."

Then the doctor said my prognosis was good because I was diagnosed young. Research showed that people who had the same characteristics as me were typically less impacted. He mentioned Betaseron again, saying it was an interferon beta drug that improved the integrity of the blood brain barrier (BBB) that has been penetrated in MS patients. He said the drug reduced the frequency of attacks by about a third, but there were side effects, such as flu-like symptoms that usually went away after the first few injections. He also mentioned I would need to be monitored for liver damage and that there might be an injection-site reaction.

"I need to give myself a shot?"

"Yes, you inject yourself every other day. What do you think?"

I wasn't ready to change my life. The shot threatened my perfect plans.

"Are there any other treatment options?"

"Betaseron is the only drug on the market that shows efficacy at reducing attacks."

I sat in silence while he continued.

"The course of action I recommend is to take the drug. It holds the best chance of reducing the impact of the disease on your body."

I wasn't convinced, based on the few facts I had gathered: doctors aren't sure what causes MS, and they aren't sure how to cure it; there is a drug that slows its progression, but I would need to inject it several times a week. The best news was that I probably had the least severe type of MS. I concluded it was best for me to live with the disease for a while to understand how it affected me before I took anything.

"Thanks for your time and your insights. I think I'm going to wait for now. See how it is living with it first."

I know my reaction to the doctor's advice was cold and probably naïve, but I was confused, angry, and in a hurry. I was defiant in my denial of the diagnosis. I wasn't ready to give in to taking the medication and was anxious to get on with my life.

My parents arrived that weekend with a surprise. Pete had flown in from Colorado and it meant so much that he was there. That afternoon we rode out to my aunt's place on the north shore of Boston and I told them about the drug. I didn't mention that I would need to inject myself a few times per week to administer it because I wasn't ready to open up discussion on whether I planned to take it.

Pete wanted to know if Betaseron was a cure. I reiterated what Dr. Book had told me and I tried to keep the conversation upbeat by sharing Dr. Book's optimism—science was moving fast and a cure could be around the corner.

My mom then asked the question I hoped to avoid.

"Are you going to take the drug?"

"I don't think so. I want to live with the disease so I can understand how it affects me, and I want to do some more research before I start giving myself a shot."

My mom didn't agree with my hesitancy; she vehemently believed I needed to take the drug. She had taken lithium for the past twenty years to manage her bi-polar disorder. I realized resistance was futile; a mother concerned about the welfare of her child would not yield, so I gave in.

"Mom, I'll think about it."

End of discussion. For now. As we drove through the North Shore, we passed the street where my father lived in high school. It was nice to be with family in familiar surroundings. Even though I felt comfortable, I didn't open up. The last thing I wanted to do was engage my own negative emotions, so I hid my turmoil with upbeat small talk.

However, by Saturday afternoon, Pete and I drove out to Crane's Beach just north of Marblehead to talk. The Crane estate, a beautiful 1920s era mansion, sat on a bluff above the beach with expansive lawns that opened to the ocean.

As we walked to the beach, I told Pete that I probably had the least severe type of MS. I assured him that because my condition had improved a lot since the episode on the basketball court, my body obviously responded well to attacks and was able to recover. There was no reason not to finish graduate school, no reason I couldn't heal completely, like I had from the optic neuritis the year prior.

"I hope to live a great life like Dr. Heller suggested," I said, adding that I didn't want to slow down. I wanted to start my company with Matt or take a job with Sapient if they made an offer, earn a black belt, get married, and have a family some day.

"Those are big aspirations," Pete said.

"That's the plan."

I returned to Cambridge after our weekend at my aunt's and made good on my promise to my mom—I did more research. I read that Betaseron was recommended because it reduced the frequency of MS episodes 20-30 percent, which was significant.

I viewed my situation optimistically. I had almost completely recovered from my attack on the basketball court. I had resumed formal classes in Tae Kwon Do and could land accurate and strong punches and kicks from my left side. If I was on a path to experience an attack every third year, Betaseron might reduce that to once every four years. Then I took a less hopeful perspective. If I was on a path to experience three episodes a year, taking the drug might reduce the frequency by one attack.

Was it worth the trouble of injecting myself a few times per week, week after week for months when my body did a good job repairing the damage on its own? It didn't seem like it.

I read more, discovering that MS could affect a person's mobility, sense of touch, strength, sight, speech, and it could cause incontinence. I also learned MS typically didn't impact a person's cognitive function, which reassured me. If the other effects occurred, I could still rely on my capacity to think. At the end of the day, there were a number of ways the disease could impact me. None of them were certain, but they were all bad.

I just wanted to continue my current lifestyle, and why couldn't I? My body seemed effective at repairing damage from an attack. I took good care of my health. I had been a vegetarian for three years. I didn't drink much alcohol. I didn't smoke. I rode my bike to school every day, and I worked out at least three times each week. I would not inject myself and would proceed on my path: graduate, get a good job, make a lot of money, live a great life—oh, and ignore MS.

After my long day of research, I stopped at the health food store around the corner from my apartment to pick up dinner, needing something more nutritious than a pizza. As I waited for my order, I browsed some displayed reading material on healthy living. I picked two books, one on detoxifying the body, called *The Colon Health Handbook*, the other titled *Enzyme Nutrition*. The books seemed to hold great insight on healthy living that would benefit me in light of my diagnosis so I bought them and took them home.

I read as I ate. The books made a lot of sense but seemed extreme. I would have to make significant lifestyle changes to follow the advice. Raw food? Are you kidding me? I loved food, even healthy food, but I liked it cooked. The thought of eating nothing but nuts and leafy green vegetables for the rest of my life left me depressed. I craved chili rellenos, an occasional beer, a slice of chocolate cake, cheese, and a good glass of wine.

Raw food was the last thing I considered as an alternative to taking Betaseron, or any other drug for that matter. I honored my vow of minimalism. Less is more, right? Why complicate my life with all this alternative stuff? The disease hadn't impacted me very much, and truth be told, I didn't want to put in all the work.

I had a great life to live and didn't want to be inconvenienced. I closed the books and put them on a shelf where they would remain for another eight years. Little did I know that they held the key to saving my life.

2

HIDING BEHIND THE WOODPILE

I took my first vows as a five-and-a half-year-old behind the single-story, chocolate-colored home where I lived with my family in a quiet neighborhood in northwestern Vermont. My father managed the production of armaments at the General Electric plant in Burlington, and my mom stayed at home and raised Pete and me. I loved having a big brother. I was glued to his hip as we sledded down snow-covered hills in winter, dammed the streams swollen with snow melt in spring, searched the woods for salamanders in summer, and jumped in leaf piles in fall.

It was mostly an ideal existence, until one night in October, 1975, when I was five; my mom rustled my brother and me out of bed at two in the morning in the freezing cold.

"Hurry boys, hurry, they're coming, they're going to get us! We must go right now! The *Mafia* is coming! Hurry!"

As we ran past the entry closet, my mom grabbed my heavy winter jacket. I struggled with the zipper while we dashed out the door. The cold drove fear into my bones as I scurried across the sidewalk.

Though only five, I knew about the Mafia from watching TV. I didn't know much about them, but I knew enough to be scared.

"Colette, where are you going? Back in the house!" My dad yelled as he appeared at the front door.

Pete listened to my dad and followed my mom back into the house, but I bolted. I ran into the backyard. I wasn't going to let the Mafia get me. It was pitch black, and the glow from our neighbor's house guided me. I frantically looked for a place to hide. I scooted behind the woodpile and gasped for air.

Behind the woodpile, I buried my face in my arms and cried. My heart pounded as I struggled to regain my breath. Thoughts raced through my head. Was I safe behind the woodpile? Was the Mafia going to shoot my parents and brother dead? If the Mafia did kill them, I knew I'd be on my own.

I told myself: *You need to be strong and take care of yourself to stay safe.*

As I remained hidden, I heard the sound of sirens grow louder. Then I saw lights flash in the front yard and summoned the courage to peek from behind the woodpile as an ambulance pulled into our driveway. The siren lights cast shadows on the neighbors who stood in our side yard. When I saw the ambulance and the neighbors gathered, I figured it was okay to leave the safety of my hideout, so I cautiously made my way.

As I turned the corner and walked across the driveway, I heard the crackle of voices on the ambulance walkie-talkie. I walked toward the front porch and stopped, wide-eyed and incredulous as I watched two paramedics cart my mom from the house on a stretcher, while a third paramedic administered oxygen.

Was she okay? Did something happen as I ran behind the house, or did the Mafia somehow get her while I was hidden?

I stood in shock at the front door, when my dad appeared. He usually didn't express emotion verbally. His face revealed his feelings. We referred to them as "looks" in later years. As my dad followed my mom out the front door, I grabbed his leg. I remember I felt safe clinging to him. I looked up and asked, "Dad, what's wrong with Mom?"

My dad looked down. "Jon, I'm not sure what's wrong, but these nice people are going to take her to the hospital and make sure she's okay."

I wanted to believe him. I wanted to believe that we would all be okay.

◆

The next morning, Pete and I watched cartoons. Later, after we finished our cereal, my dad came in and joined us. He clicked off the TV and sat in his chair.

"Your mom is sick and will probably be in the hospital for a bit, but she wanted me to make sure you know she misses and loves you both very much."

"What's wrong with her?" Pete asked.

"The doctors aren't sure, so they're going to run some tests."

"Really?" I said, full of disappointment.

My mind raced through the days ahead. I had just started kindergarten, and mom helped me get ready for school each day. I suddenly became anxious. Who would help me get dressed and make my lunch?

I heard the vow again. *You need to be strong and take care of yourself to stay safe.* I wanted to cry but didn't. I concealed my fear and anger to show how strong I was.

My dad said that my Aunt Sue would arrive for a visit on Sunday afternoon to help around the house until Mom came home. I was excited to see Aunt Sue; she was stricter than my mom, but we always had fun.

Then Dad's face turned serious.

"Boys, there's something I need to tell you."

Pete and I moved closer.

"It's best you don't talk about what happened last night," my father said, as if he was instructing us in how to fix a leaky bike tire. This was

1975, after all, and mental health disorders were not something that anyone we knew spoke of freely. "If other people ask how your mother is, say she's doing better and that she will probably be home in a couple of weeks."

I turned away and stared at the empty TV screen. A couple of weeks? How long was that? It seemed like forever. I didn't know if I had the endurance to keep all this inside me, but I would slowly learn how to become a master at keeping secrets: first my mother's bi-polar condition, and later my own condition; they were good reasons to keep tight-lipped in the future and protect my family.

3

GO WITH SAPIENT

A week after the diagnosis, Sapient offered me a job as an assistant project manager. I was thrilled. I wanted to begin my career with a fast-growing, well-respected company and Sapient appeared to provide a rapid climb up the corporate ladder.

My future compensation would be a mix of cash and stock options. I had the potential to get rich, very rich, if the company continued to grow at the same rate it had in each of its first six years. I wanted to develop my skills and contribute to its growth. Growing rich had suddenly become very important to me. Ever since the diagnosis, I assumed an urgency to become financially independent. I had no idea how long I would be able to work—maybe two years, maybe twenty. I knew I didn't want to rely on anyone to bail me out of my situation. This was my problem, and I would find a way to handle it on my own. Just like I handled "the Mafia" of my childhood.

I accepted the offer and called my parents to share the good news. My mom answered.

"I just received a call from Sapient, and they offered me a job ssistant project manager in their San Francisco office," I gushed.

'on, that's wonderful, I'm so happy for you," my mom said.

'e thing."

"What's that?"

"Please don't tell anyone about the diagnosis. I don't want people to judge me and for it to potentially impact my advancement. I don't have any idea how the disease will impact me. There's a chance I may never have another attack. Can you keep my secret?"

"Sure, honey," my mom said hesitantly and passed the phone to my dad.

"Dad, Sapient offered me a job in San Francisco as an assistant project manager."

"Great. When do you start?"

"September 1. I'll need another couple of months to finish my thesis, and then I'll pack my things to move west."

The line went silent while my dad considered the gravity of what I had just shared. He usually was one or two steps ahead, but not this time. I had just been diagnosed with a serious illness and now planned to move three thousand miles away.

I knew he was happy for me, but his silence revealed a new level of concern. Right before I hung up, I repeated my request to not mention the diagnosis to anyone. "Your secret is safe," he said, and I trusted him, knowing he had asked the same of Pete and me twenty years earlier.

The hardest part about accepting my job at Sapient was telling Matt. I didn't want to disappoint him after everything we had already done for our start-up, Virtual View, but I knew I had to get more practical about my future in light of the diagnosis. I believed that taking a job with a more established company, even one as young as Sapient, was a more secure bet than breaking out on my own—with Matt or anyone.

I worked up the nerve to tell him one morning after a class and went to the computer lab hoping to see Matt checking email. I made my way through the row of monitors and spotted him in the back.

"Hey Man, how's your morning?" I said in a hushed voice.

"Okay, I just reviewed the email reminder from the department about thesis dates and need to pick up the pace; how was your morning?" he whispered.

"Class was good, but I need to talk when you get a chance."

"Sure, I'll have a minute after I finish my mail. I'll come get you."

I took a seat, anxiously staring at the screen, fretting about the friendship that might unravel—all because of the MS. My stomach felt tight and I wondered if this might be the beginning of the end of my unfettered optimism. I had always been a loyal friend and, consciously or not, I regretted that the MS was making me choose otherwise.

A few minutes later, Matt tapped me on the shoulder.

"Let's step outside," I said.

We walked out into the hall. "Remember the Sapient interview I had the other week?" I asked, getting right to it. "They got back to me and offered me a position."

I expected Matt to be taken aback by my latest news, but he stood there and smiled. "I'm happy for you Jon. Tell me about it," he said as if he already knew.

When I told him about the offer and the relocation to San Francisco, he assured me that he would continue with his vision because he still fully believed in it.

"I've got the incorporation papers together, and I'll file them in the next couple of weeks," he said.

I was finally able to breathe.

"I'm really sorry that I won't be able to work with you," I said. "I think we make a great team, but I need something with... a little more certainty and security."

"I get it," Matt said and caught my eye. "You have to do what you have to do."

4

MOVING TO THE EDGE ON THE WEST COAST

In the summer of 1997 I finished my thesis, received my diploma, and graduated from MIT. I had healed completely from the episode on the basketball court. My limp was gone, and I was in total control of my left hand and leg as evidenced by accurate punches and kicks at Tae Kwan Do. I was moving to a great city to start work at a great company. I was living my dream, and it had no room for multiple sclerosis.

Though my parents and Pete supported my decision to keep quiet about the diagnosis, I knew I was asking a lot. Later, I realized I was denying them the kind of support that might also have helped me heal. At the time, I wanted to spare myself and others the grim consequences of MS—a life of increased paralysis that progressed from the use of a cane to a walker to a wheelchair. That was not my idea of a great life. Besides, I didn't know for sure how the disease would impact me; there was no reason not to be optimistic. Maybe I was one of the lucky ones.

When I arrived in San Francisco, I moved in with my friend Liz, a classmate from MIT, who lived in Oakland. I planned to live on her couch for a few weeks until I found a place. It was an exciting time to arrive—those were the early days of the dot-com boom, and the Bay Area was the epicenter. I was living my teenage aspirations.

In my teens, I remember waiting each summer for my dad to receive Forbes magazine's annual list of the top-paid CEOs for the five hundred largest public companies, America's captains of industry. After my dad finished reading it, I would take it up to my bedroom and study it. More than anything, I wanted to be on that list.

From my first day at Sapient, I was eager to work hard, build a strong reputation, and gain responsibility. I wanted to be perceived as a go-getter, hungry to take on new challenges and prove to myself that MS wasn't going to impact me. I worked hard to exceed client and team expectations on each project. I wanted to show I was a vital team contributor who helped achieve high levels of client satisfaction.

As a result, I was offered an opportunity to lead the testing phase of a project in Los Angeles. I joined a team of young, bright, and highly motivated software developers in their twenties who worked their butts off to prove their mettle. Thirty of us were sequestered in a cramped forty-by-forty-foot room in the old Playboy call center at the west end of LA's San Fernando Valley writing code for a start-up online insurance agency, AFI. The atmosphere was collegiate; we worked hard and played hard.

We turned the InFocus projector, used to deliver client presentations, into a movie projector on Friday nights to watch action movies on the side of the building after dark. We hung out on weekends, drinking beer at local bars, and ran touch football tournaments in an empty back parking lot during lunch.

But it wasn't all fun and games; it was my responsibility to make sure the application we were developing was built, as designed, and that it worked—all while keeping my darkest secret from everyone, fearing it might jeopardize my success.

♦

In the summer of 1998, the AFI application went live, and Sapient opened a Los Angeles office, leveraging the team to build its talent. Frank Schettino, the managing director of the office, approached me and offered me a position as one of the founding members of the LA staff. I jumped at the opportunity. The company's growth strategy challenged current employees to fill open jobs from within; providing a tangible ladder to climb.

Frank and I had gone to lunch my first month on the job in San Francisco. He told me to deliver on my commitments, become an expert at what I did, and the rest would take care of itself. Though he was only a year older than me, he had been with the company for four years and had quickly risen from working the front desk to director. I knew if I watched him closely and emulated his actions, I had the opportunity to achieve the same success. If I gave work everything I had, I knew I might eventually find myself on Forbes' captains of industry list. I was on my way to realizing my dream.

5

FEED THE MACHINE

As I worked to add new products to the AFI system, I met a guy named Kelly Harriger who wrote marketing copy for the start-up. He was ten years older and an avid hiker, climber, and mountain biker. During breaks, I would stop by his desk and excitedly share stories of my weekend rides in the Santa Monica Mountains, hoping to impress him, and he told me about new trails.

Kelly had lived in LA for eight years and had biked throughout the Santa Monica and San Gabrielle Mountains. Kelly had also hiked numerous 14,000-foot peaks in the Sierras and had rock climbed noted Southern California peaks, from the famous walls of Tahquitz to the climber's paradise in Joshua Tree. I wanted to join his expeditions.

My body had shown no evidence of the symptoms that lead to the diagnosis. I didn't have any hint of a limp and hadn't had any bouts of stiffness or lack of sensation. As far as I was concerned, there was no MS. In the spring of 1999, I began to ride and hike with Kelly on the weekends. He became my outdoor mentor and introduced me to mountaineering. That summer, together with Kelly, I reached the top of my first 14,000-foot Sierra summit, Split Mountain, and began a quest to climb each of the thirteen fourteen-thousand-foot Sierra peaks. I hoped my drive to push beyond my limits would prove the MS didn't exist. There was certainly no reason to tell Kelly my secret.

I believed my body was a machine and continued to work eighty hours, for weeks on end. I thought that if I stayed in good physical condition, my body would be strong enough to withstand anything—the hours, the miles, even the MS. I pushed myself hard, and took food for granted. My default meals were chili relleno, a bean and cheese burrito, or a cheese pizza. I just needed to feed my body calories to function, like the Energizer Bunny. It didn't matter what kind as long as I had a mix of fats, carbohydrates, and proteins. It would take me time to learn that not all calories were the same, and that health was more than just being physically fit—but that was a lesson for another day.

Saturday morning was the only time I didn't work. I rode my bike instead. One morning, as Kelly and I rode past the pier on our way to the Santa Monica Mountains, I was struck by the stillness. Since I spent so much time working, I hadn't developed other hobbies or interests that encouraged introspection. I rationalized that the long work hours were worth the sacrifice, to build my career and accumulate the money I might someday need if the MS ever immobilized me.

As we rode to the trailhead, we headed inland from the beach and passed multi-million-dollar estates. I wanted to live in one of those homes because it would prove I had "made it," the level of success I told myself I needed to achieve to live a great life.

After the initial thousand-foot climb, the road turned from the affluent suburban neighborhood into a wilderness trail, and the grade increased significantly. As I climbed, my legs and lungs burned, but I was pleased—my body seemed to be in top shape. I felt no effects of MS. Was I beating the diagnosis? I loved how present I felt during bike rides—the cadence of each pedal stroke and each deep, cleansing breath cleared the chaos from my mind and brought greater balance.

We arrived at a bluff that overlooked the Santa Monica Bay. I paused to catch my breath and take in the dramatic sights of a completely unpopulated mountain. The terrain was covered in lush green vegetation.

I looked over at Kelly and said, "Wow, hard to believe this is LA."

We hopped on our bikes and continued the climb. The trail's pitch steepened even more, and it took all of my attention to navigate the rocky route. I dug deeper to concentrate and keep my momentum. After several miles of a steep uphill grind, the trail evened out, and we reached Mulholland Drive. I stopped to rest and soak in the serenity. I felt great. This was as close to a perfect moment as I could imagine. I was pleased to have put my body through the intense workout and, more importantly, that my body met the challenge. I was ready to bomb back to the beach and glanced at my watch.

"Kelly, we rode fourteen miles and gained 2,500 feet in an hour and a half. How'd we do?

"That's fast."

"How fast?"

"Real fast."

I felt good, knowing I had probably ridden the trail faster than any previous morning during the past six months. I was hoping for stronger validation of our performance, but that was the extent of Kelly's emotional expression. As much as I wanted more, I appreciated his cool, even-keeled response.

We mounted our bikes to finish the ride. As we started down the trail, Kelly asked what I planned to do after the ride.

"Not much."

"What do you think about stopping by my buddy Brendan's place?"

"Cool."

I had heard a lot about Brendan. He had climbed several 14ers (14,000-foot peaks) with Kelly, and I was eager to meet him. I hoped our introduction might bring me closer to climbing those mountains myself.

We flew down the hill and were back in the middle of Santa Monica by ten o'clock. We parked our bikes behind Brendan's place.

"Hey bud, you there?" Kelly yelled, as we stepped through his back gate.

"Yep, be right there. I need to get something."

Suddenly Brendan appeared. He was six-two, long and lean.

"What's up, dude?" He said, as he looked at Kelly and gave me a glance.

"This is my buddy, Chando."

"Hey man," Brendan said, with the cocksure coolness of a rock star.

"Hey," I shot back, wondering what he'd done to injure his face. Brendan's mouth and front lip looked like they had been fed through a sausage grinder.

"Is that what happened last weekend?" Kelly asked.

"Yep, endo'd and bit a rock up on backbone."

I would come to learn later the "backbone trail" was one of the most extreme rides in the Santa Monica Mountains.

"I just bought this new helmet."

Brendan held it out for us to inspect. It was a full-face helmet and looked like the ones BMX racers wore. "The dental work to repair the tooth was ridiculous! Got the helmet so I don't have to shell out more cash if I go over the handle bars again."

We talked a little while longer, and then Kelly got itchy. "Well dude, we need to get home, got some things to take care of. Maybe we can ride next weekend," Kelly said as he turned to leave.

I had learned over the previous six months that Kelly wasn't one to hang around. It was similar to how he rode—impatient but efficient.

"Great idea, let's do it!" Brendan replied.

♦

The next morning, I woke and grabbed some breakfast, anticipating the ride Kelly had invited me on with Brendan the next weekend. I loved being included but was anxious about Brendan and Kelly finding out about my secret. I wanted them to see me as they saw themselves—in top physical condition, ready for any adventure. What I really needed was not just their invitation for companionship; I needed them to witness how much the MS wasn't affecting me. If I could hang with them, I couldn't be *that* ill.

I decided to train for my ride with Brendan and Kelly on a trail near the Jet Propulsion Laboratory in Pasadena. I parked, unloaded my bike, threw on my Camelback, and headed up the trail, riding the 2,500-foot, eight-mile ascent in about forty minutes.

After the climb, the trail evened out before descending again. As I began to pick up speed on the downhill, my front tire bottomed out in a gully and nearly caused me to fly over the handlebars. I was able to hold on, and at the last second, my momentum carried me and the bike through the obstacle.

However, as I continued to bomb downhill, a tree suddenly appeared in the middle of the trail and forced me to swerve. I turned hard to the right and into the mountain, because the trail dropped sharply to the left. I overcorrected and watched my front tire go horizontal across the trail's centerline in the direction of a ravine. This time I couldn't correct myself and flew off my bike and down an embankment, falling forty feet and landing on my back in a drainage ditch.

A pile of leaves and vines cushioned my fall. Luckily, my bike had stayed on the trail above and hadn't landed on top of me. As I lay on my back, I wasn't sure what happened. I looked up through the trees and saw brilliant blue sky and heard birds sing. I could see and hear, so I was conscious. I scanned my body and felt no immediate pain.

I sat and looked up at the embankment. That's when I realized I was in trouble. My mind raced, wondering how I would ever make it out, when I spotted the metal rungs of a ladder encased in the concrete retaining wall. I stood up and started to climb, thinking how lucky I was to get out of the ravine without injury.

When I got back on the trail, I checked my bike for damage. The spokes checked out, but the chain was off the derailleur. I put the chain back on, climbed on my bike, and slowly started down the trail, suddenly disturbed. Had I crashed because I was riding too fast, or because I was in the midst of an MS attack?

One Sunday that summer, I asked Frank to go on a mountain bike ride. I wanted to hang out, but what I really wanted to do was to share my secret. I didn't expect anything to happen as the result of telling him. I definitely didn't want him to feel sorry for me. I just wanted him to know about the diagnosis in case I became impacted by symptoms later on down the road. If my worst fear came true, I didn't want to catch him off guard or for him to be taken by surprise. I wanted our relationship to have a solid foundation of trust. About half an hour into our ride, I pulled up to Frank's back wheel and began my confession. "I love these flat sections, they cause me to lose myself in the ride and forget about the stresses of the past week at work."

"It's great up here. You would never know we were a few miles from LA with all these green mountains around us. Do you ride up here often?" he said.

"I come up here every Saturday and some Sundays."

"I'm impressed with all of your running and riding, Jon. You're in great shape. I remember you used to walk to work each morning when the team was working on the AFI project. I commend you for your commitment to being healthy."

"There's a reason I work so hard to stay in shape."

"What's that?" he asked.

There. We had hit the perfect segue and I took a deep breath.

"I have MS."

There was a long pause while we both stopped pedaling and coasted, so Frank could digest what I had said.

"WOW . . . MS, huh . . . I had no idea."

"You know what it is, right?"

"Multiple sclerosis. I know someone who has it but who doesn't take care of himself like you do."

"I work so hard to stay fit because I want to do everything I can to work a long prosperous career," I said, looking off into the canyon.

"That's a good goal; let's hope that's the case," he said.

6

RUN, RUN ... AS FAST AS YOU CAN

At the start of the millennium, I was firing on all cylinders. My drive for success and decision to deny the diagnosis were working, at least from all appearances. I set goals and earned a strong reputation at Sapient, while building a solid nest egg. Physically, I was invincible. I rode with Brendan and Kelly on weekends and sometimes during the week after work. I even joined their quest to climb the fourteen thousand foot Sierra peaks. Fortune was shining on me—big and bright. I had lived the last three years without a hint of MS symptoms, and I hoped my good fortune would continue.

Instead of allowing my fear of MS to slow me down, it had the opposite effect. It propelled me to make the most of every moment. Though I had run before, I had only done so to train for a sport in school. I started again because I liked the sensation of strength, the feeling of freedom, and the high from the endorphin surge. Running complimented the biking and helped me stay in shape. I had never run for the sake of running, but I now ran because I knew one day I might not even be able to walk.

◆

One night after a run, I grabbed dinner at my favorite Mexican joint, Holy Guacamole, where I always ate at the counter. I had no one to go home to and wanted to be around other people. It upset me to eat alone, but it was a conscious choice. I felt that if I were in a relationship that I might have to share my time between my athletic and professional goals and the needs of being in harmony with a woman. The thought scared the hell out of me. I might not be able to strike the balance and wouldn't be successful in either. Most of all, I was terrified I wouldn't be able to maintain my health.

I waited for my food and took out my athletic journal to pass the time—entering the distance, duration, and elevation gained from my weekend rides and my run that night. My meal arrived, and I took out a book, *4 Months to a 4-Hour Marathon,* by Dave Kuehls, to read while I ate. The uncertainty of the disease's progression lurked in the back of my mind, but based on the book's approach, I had enough time to train for the LA marathon that spring. I felt a marathon would be my next great physical test, which I believed was keeping the MS at bay. And I didn't plan to just finish; I wanted to cross the line in under three hours and thirty minutes, the qualifying time for the Boston Marathon.

The next day, I went to work full of excitement about my marathon goal and pulled aside the assistant project manager, Brock Meltzer. He had just joined the company that summer, so we had known each other for only a few months but were becoming fast friends. I knew he was a runner and was looking for a training partner.

"I put together a plan to run the LA marathon in March. Want to run it together?"

"Yeah, sure, I'm in!" he said without a hint of hesitation.

I liked Brock's decisiveness. We committed to running every Sunday and occasionally during the week. I loved running with him. It was good to talk about work, but it was more than that—Brock motivated me to train, to stay in top shape, to have a shot at qualifying for the Boston Marathon, and to hopefully out-run the MS.

At the end of a long run one Sunday morning, we reached Hill Street and raced to my apartment. My legs and lungs burned, but it felt good to push myself, knowing that my body was still there for me. As I relaxed on my couch afterward, I calculated our performance. We had run twelve miles, almost a half-marathon, and had run a seven-minute-and-forty-five-second mile pace—the pace we needed to complete the marathon in three hours and thirty minutes. It was fast, but my body felt good.

The big day arrived. Brock and I ran stride for stride for the first thirteen miles, when I realized I needed to pick up the pace if I wanted to qualify for Boston. I accelerated ahead of Brock, then realized I had probably taken it too far. When I hit the wall at mile twenty-two, my pace slowed considerably, and I was alone. I dug deep, moved to the side of the course, and pushed myself to the end. I finished in three hours and forty-six minutes and missed the time to qualify for Boston by sixteen minutes. My slower pace wasn't on account of the MS; I was like any other novice marathon runner who hit the wall after running twenty-two miles.

I was thankful to have completed the run and finish a marathon, but I wondered if I might have reached my goal to qualify for Boston if I'd stayed with Brock. He had finished a few minutes behind me, but I asked myself if we had run the last half of the race together, whether we might have been able to motivate each other to run faster. I was startled by a realization. I was not good at considering another person's goal in relation to my own, especially if it threatened my secret in any way. Regrettably, my impulse to outrun the MS would cost me companionship, but I wasn't ready to face that demon yet.

7

A TEXAS PRISON AND A GAME-CHANGING HAIRCUT

Six weeks after I finished the marathon, I walked into my boss's office, took a seat, and discussed the opportunity I had been offered with the prison project in Huntsville, Texas.

"You know about the project's past?" Frank began.

I was no stranger to the tone. It was the one my father used any time I was about to dive into a huge challenge: caution buffered by optimism.

"I spoke with Chris and Michael about their experiences," I said, trying to reassure him and myself. "I look forward to the challenge."

Frank nodded. "Do you know you will be responsible for delivering the testing phase?"

"I do. I look forward to working with the client to confirm the system is ready to go live."

"And you know that it will be a bigger challenge than usual because of the project's history?"

I looked Frank in the eye. He was clearly testing me.

"I look forward to it," I said.

"You know it's at least a six- to nine-month commitment, maybe longer?"

"I do."

"Any questions or concerns?"

"I'll be able to fly back to LA on weekends, right?"

"You will need to confirm that with project leadership."

Frank had given me every chance to explore whether it was the right opportunity, but I didn't take it. This was my first venture into the arena of troubled projects. I didn't ask any questions because I didn't know the right ones to ask, and I didn't want my questions to cause Frank to second-guess if I was up to the challenge. Denial continued to blind me, and I looked past the project's troubled past the same way I looked past the diagnosis, believing that I could take on any challenge and end up on top.

Two weeks later, I boarded a flight to Houston for what would become a weekly ritual for the next fourteen months. We were building a system for the Texas Department of Criminal Justice to track offenders after they were released and put on parole. Several colleagues who had returned to Santa Monica after serving their time in Texas dubbed it "the prison project." Since I wasn't staffed to a project and was 'on the bench,' a common phrase in the world of consulting, I was available to any team that needed me and was called on to help finish the project. I was excited about the opportunity.

I landed in Houston and drove a hundred miles north to Huntsville. My second night in town, I moved into a corporate apartment, and the reality of my decision to be staffed there hit home. While the project had benefits, it had a downside. The locals were not fond of "tree-huggin' Californians," and I had trouble finding anything vegetarian on the menus, though I was amazed at all of the creative ways bacon could be used.

There were also professional challenges. I knew the Texas prison application was large and complex. I knew the previous team had difficulty wrapping up the design, but the team eventually completed the phase, and the project continued. I found out that one of the contractors on the project had been sued by the State of Texas. The state's famed motto, *don't mess with Texas*, was a threat that lingered over the project and reinforced my own: *be strong and take care of yourself to stay safe*. Nothing was going to mess with me in Texas. Not our client, not the prison, and certainly not MS.

I hoped to orient myself to Huntsville by re-establishing my fitness routine. On several nights after work that first week, I left my apartment in search of a four-mile training course. I planned to race in the Pier to Peak half-marathon and Malibu Triathlon that summer and the Philadelphia Marathon that fall. The Pier to Peak race may have seemed easy after I had just completed a full marathon two months earlier; the challenge was running up a 4,000 foot mountain.

The Nautica Malibu Triathlon would be my first triathlon and was considered short in the world of triathlons: a half-mile ocean swim, eighteen-mile road-ride, and four-mile run. I had the ride and run covered. My weekend rides in the mountains and training runs after work would prepare me for those legs. The difficulty of a triathlon would be the swim and transitioning between the three events. I was most concerned about the swim. I had quit the swim team at the age of ten, twenty-one years earlier, because I didn't like the water. I would need to find a pool in Huntsville to train after work on the nights I didn't run. I would also need to overcome my fear of the water, but that was no big deal. I had the denial thing nailed.

To keep things simple, I focused on running. All I had to do was throw on my running shoes and hit the road. One night, my course took me through the center of town, which consisted of one square block of shops and restaurants. As I reached the run's halfway point and decided to return to my apartment, I headed down what appeared to be a rarely traveled side street. A few hundred yards later, a large imposing brick wall appeared in the distance that first looked like the outer wall of a fortress. Then it struck me—I was staring at the outer wall of the prison.

I turned and ran home, thankful to be a free man, but my mind never strayed from that huge wall, even when I was at work.

I flew back to LA from Texas every Friday night, eager to ride with Kelly and Brendan on the weekends and run along the beach. On my eighth trip home, my plan was the same, but when I opened up my mailbox—I discovered a letter from my mother. I recognized her handwriting immediately. I eagerly went upstairs and found a place on the couch to relax and savor the letter. She caught me up on their news then turned serious.

I sometimes wonder if you're lonely, if you are steering away from a relationship with a woman because of the MS. Any woman worth her salt would love to spend her life with you. Of course, I am a slightly prejudiced mom, but seriously, Jon, please don't let the MS keep you from loving someone.

I put the letter down. I was shocked that my mother could see the reality of my existence so clearly, and it hurt to be seen like this. I wanted to be the strong son; the successful son. Not the sick and frail son. She saw beyond my mask, and her words struck me harder than I thought imaginable. My mom was right. I had chosen to be alone, and I didn't have anyone to greet me when I returned from my ride, or to share my intimate thoughts or my Texas troubles with. But there was a good reason. My first priority was my career. I wanted to develop a solid professional foundation in order to build a solid financial foundation while staying in top physical condition. Couldn't my mother see that the only relationship I could afford to focus on was with myself?

I wanted to tell her that independence—from my parents and everyone else, was my idea of living a great life, but as I sat on my couch with the letter in hand, I thought about all I had accomplished during the previous four years. I was living the "Great Life" I envisioned for myself, but I couldn't help but think there was something missing.

If I had no one to share this so-called great life with, what was the point?

◆

I needed a haircut and called the hair salon around the corner on Main Street to schedule an appointment. As much as I tried to ignore it, my mother's letter had an impact, and I followed her advice. I had a mad crush on my stylist, Robyn, and asked for an appointment that afternoon. I knew I might not be able to get one because I was calling so late. Robyn was talented and her schedule filled up fast, but I got lucky. She had a cancellation that afternoon.

Before I walked out the door, I grabbed *The Four Agreements* by Miguel Ruiz, the book Robyn lent me after our last appointment. She had told me she was reading a great book and thought I'd like it too. I asked to borrow it, hoping to impress her, and read the book during my next four flights back and fourth to Texas. If this was her way of probing my values, it was a great test. Did she want to know if I honored the 'four agreements' in my daily life? Be Impeccable With Your Words, Don't Take Anything Personally, Don't Make Assumptions, and Always Do Your Best. In recommending the book to me, Robyn had inadvertently revealed a lot about herself, and I loved every bit.

I carried the book down the hill to Ambiance Salon, enjoying the short walk to Main Street. It reminded me of the small-town street shopping districts in the main-line suburbs of Philadelphia and Fairfield County, Connecticut, where I lived during middle and high school. I felt the refreshing ocean breeze as I walked and had a skip in my step. I felt like I was home and looked forward to spending time with Robyn, even if it was only for a half-hour haircut.

I walked into the salon, took a seat on the couch, and waited. I was nervous. I felt like it was the first time I was seeing her, even though she'd cut my hair every month for the previous year. I was particular about my hair—it was unruly and not just any stylist could cut it right, but my anxiety had nothing to do with Robyn's skills. I was anxious in her presence. Not exactly the cool cat I had hoped to be.

I watched as she finished with her current client and admired her from afar. I was very attracted to her physically. She stood about five foot six in her sexy, open-toed high-healed shoes. She had blond hair, blue eyes, and a great body. She walked her client to the door and said good-bye. My heart jumped. It was my turn, and I was smitten. She walked toward me on the couch. I stood and she gave me a hug. I probably embraced her longer than I should have.

"How are you?" she asked.

"I'm good. I'm home for the weekend. I read that book you lent me," I said as I walked to her chair.

I sat and handed her *The Four Agreements*.

"What did you think?" she asked, as she placed it on her station.

"Great book, he's a good writer."

That was the extent of my expression. I was too emotionally illiterate to share my feelings. She knew it and let me slide.

She focused on my hair. "Did you like what I did last time?"

"It was perfect. Short on the sides, and leave the top a little longer."

"I know," she said with a hint of enthusiasm.

She was good at her craft and knew how I liked it. She handed me a smock and showed me to the dressing room. I walked out and she led me to the sink. When she rubbed shampoo into my hair, I could feel her fingers massage my scalp. The warm water and her touch relaxed me. I sat with my head under the water and my eyes shut in a state of bliss. When she finished, I followed her back to her chair, where she toweled the water from my hair and combed it out. I didn't want her hands to leave me.

"I always forget how curly your hair is," she said with a smile.

"Yeah, the water runs right off it like a Brillo Pad."

I watched her in the mirror as we both laughed. Her easy laugh relaxed me.

"How was your week?" she asked.

"I spent the week in Texas working on the prison project."

"I remember you told me about it last time. How's it going?"

"It's a lot of work. We're working long hours to rebuild client confidence, the food's not what I'm used to, and it's getting really hot, but I'm able to run, and I've found a pool to swim in after work."

"Oh wow that doesn't sound fun . . . sorry."

"No big deal. I asked for the challenge. How was your week?"

"Great."

"What was so good about it?"

"Girls' night last Sunday."

"Oh yeah? Tell me."

"Two of my really close girlfriends came over for girls night "in". We had dinner and watched Sex and the City," she said, cracking up.

"What was so funny?"

She paused and let out a nervous laugh. "Um," she giggled, "not sure you'd be interested."

I sensed her apprehension to share, but for some reason I asked.

"Tell me, what was so funny?"

"You sure you want to know?" she laughed.

Now I felt like she was trying to hide something. "Yeah, tell me."

"Well, the episode was about Samantha, you know Kim Cattrall's character, the one who's the nympho?"

"I know the show," I said. Though I worked most hours of the day, I wasn't a total social aberration. Robyn caught my eye and smiled.

"Okay, so Samantha had had it with men and wanted to experience what it was like to be with another woman, so she starts a relationship with Maria. They had a fight, and Maria bought her a strap-on to make up, but Samantha tweaked her neck when they tried it out."

I watched in the mirror as Robyn rotated her head to the left and pinned her chin to her shoulder and cracked up. I totally let my guard down in Robyn's presence and couldn't remember the last time I laughed so hard. Robyn had a real gift for conversation. She made me feel at ease, even when discussing a subject that would have made me very uptight talking about with anyone else.

Before I knew it, she was finished with my haircut. Robyn looked down at her watch, realizing we had gone ten minutes over time. She peaked around the corner and saw her next appointment waiting on the couch. Our time together had run out. I'd have to wait another four weeks. She finished buzzing my neck, pulled the smock off, and I stood and walked to the counter to pay. My appointment was over, and I was bummed.

Robyn walked with me to the register. I wanted to leave the salon knowing I would see her again, so I scheduled an appointment in July. Before I turned to walk out, she gave me a hug and kissed my cheek. I glanced in the mirror and noticed she had left a red lipstick mark. She laughed nervously and wiped it off and joked, "Good luck in Texas... There's more where that came from."

I could feel my face turn crimson. I wasn't sure what she insinuated with the comment and hastily turned to leave and walked straight into the door. Crash went the shades. I looked down and quickly walked out, thinking Robyn and the other stylists were about to erupt with laughter. What an exit! At least I didn't have to worry about her forgetting about me.

When I returned to my apartment, it was too quiet. I couldn't stop thinking about Robyn and my mom's letter, even though I knew dating was potentially dangerous ground. But for some reason, I felt differently. Our discussions in her chair were more open and honest than my typical interactions with women. I was able to be myself without the enthusiastic charade I'd mastered since I'd been diagnosed.

Over the previous year, we talked about our days growing up in New England and the implications of the George W. Bush era on the country. I felt comfortable and free around her. At the end of my haircuts, I left wishing we could go to a café and spend the next couple of hours chatting over a bottle of wine. Robyn didn't strike me as the kind of person I'd need to hide from, but I decided, early on, I wasn't going to threaten our connection by telling her about the MS.

I picked up the phone and dialed the salon.

"May I please speak with Robyn?" I asked the receptionist.

"She's just finishing up with a client, please hold?"

I was in luck. If she had been too busy to talk, I would have had to call her back, and I probably would have lost my nerve. I waited for thirty seconds—what seemed like an eternity for her to answer.

"This is Robyn."

"Hey Robyn. Jon Chandonnet."

"Hey, what's up?" she replied, sounding surprised.

"You missed a spot."

"What?"

"Yeah, one of the sides isn't right."

"Seriously, I'm so sorry! Come right down, and I'll fix it," she said.

I smiled on my side of the phone. I didn't want to worry her, but she seemed confident she could fix anything.

"Actually, the haircut is great. I'm calling to see if you want to go for a drink tonight after work?"

"Huh?"

"What do you think about getting a drink after work?"

There was a pause on the other side of the line. I cringed; this was WAY outside my comfort zone. My confidence waned with every passing second.

"Um . . . I'm going rollerblading after work."

Her answer was a serious blow to my confidence, but I stayed with it. "That's cool. I'm going over to my buddy Brendan's to watch a rerun of last year's Tour de France. What do you say we get a drink at the World Café after? I'll be in the lounge."

I tried to make it easy for her to say yes.

"Well . . . I guess so," she said.
"How does eight sound?"
"Okay, eight it is."
"Great, see you then!"

PART III
THE CLIMB

8

MS CHAPERONES A FIRST DATE

Later that night, I sat in the lounge of World Café, my favorite bar on Main Street. I found a seat with a view of the entrance, so that I could see Robyn arrive, then waited anxiously for the cocktail waitress. I needed a drink and ordered a bourbon and ginger.

This was my first date in months. The diagnosis had kept me from opening up to colleagues, let alone a woman I liked. My guarded nature was nurtured, if not fully created by living under a veil of family secrets. I kept tight lipped about my mother's bi-polar condition and my MS diagnosis. I believed every word I uttered was public record and might come back to haunt me, and I debated whether or not I should tell Robyn.

The waitress arrived with my drink; I took a sip and felt immediate warmth the instant the bourbon hit my bloodstream. I looked at my watch; it was five minutes to eight. I scanned the bar to make sure Robyn hadn't come in and recognized two of her colleagues from the salon, Holli and Lora, sitting with three other women. I entertained the idea of joining them before my attention was struck by Robyn, wearing a sexy blue mini-dress walking through the café courtyard. The orange glow of the California sunset silhouetted her body. She wore an intense look on her face that I recognized from years of competitive sports: it was game time.

I stood and met her with a big hug.

"Hey, how are you?" she said with a coquettish grin.

"Wow, you look great," I said, feeling a chill radiate through me when I looked into her blue eyes. "Here, take a seat."

"Thanks."

"How was your blade?"

"So much fun! We went down towards Malibu and saw dolphins."

Robyn looked up at my hair. "How do you like your hair cut?"

"Looks great, you always do such a good job."

"I was horrified when you called and said I missed a spot."

"Sorry, I had to think of some reason other than asking you out to give you a call. I wouldn't have had the nerve otherwise."

"I've never messed up a client's haircut," she said and smiled.

"Sorry. Let me get you a drink."

"Deal, a Kettle One Martini, dirty."

I wanted to make sure Robyn was as comfortable as possible, so I mentioned that I had seen Holli and Lora from the salon with a group of friends at the bar and asked if she wanted to join them.

"Sure," she said.

We got up and moved to the bar. I found out later that my offer to sit with her friends had won me huge points. After half an hour, Robyn and I were connecting and the date was going well. I didn't want it to end.

"Would you like to get a bite to eat?" I suggested. "You must be hungry."

"Yeah, that would be great," Robyn said.

I could tell that she didn't want the night to end either, so I followed my earlier move and asked if she wanted her friends to join us—clearly they made her feel at ease.

"I'd love that, if it's okay with you," she said.

The host showed us to a table, and I ordered a bottle of wine. The conversation continued to flow. When the waiter came to take our dinner order, Robyn and I chose the same vegetarian pasta dish.

"Are you a vegetarian?" she asked.

"Yeah, I stopped eating red meat and chicken about six years ago. You?

"I stopped eating meat when I was fourteen."

"Why?" I asked.

"I didn't like the taste, and I couldn't stomach the thought of eating anything with a face."

I told her I made a commitment to eat healthier when I was working in North Carolina at my first real job after college. My days of drinking beer and eating whatever comforted me on the road had caused me to weigh nearly two hundred pounds.

"Seriously? I never would have known."

"It just didn't feel good to have all that extra weight, so I made the commitment to become vegetarian and get in shape."

"I remember you came into the salon to get a hair cut the day after you finished the LA Marathon. You told me about hitting the wall near the end. I remember you had to move to the side of the course and put your hazards on."

We both laughed. It felt so good to connect with a woman like this and I realized what a fool I had been to deny myself this pleasure simply out of fear. I couldn't resist wanting to touch her and looked around the table and saw Robyn's friends engrossed in conversation, then reached under the table and rested my hand on top of hers; she didn't pull it away. She just looked at me and smiled sweetly. When the waiter came to clear our dinner plates, Robyn's friend Holli made a call to extend the evening: "You guys wanna go to O'Brien's? I think they have a band tonight."

We paid the bill and headed across the street. It was eleven o'clock on Saturday night on Main Street in Santa Monica, still early for the late night partying crowd but we were ready for O'Brien's dance floor. I watched Robyn's hips move to the music. The bright lights flashed and the music vibrated through me, and the next thing I know, Robyn grabbed my hand and pulled me to the dance floor. I tried to keep up, but it was clear Robyn had taken dance as a kid. Her movement was infectious and fluid. The more she got into it, the harder I tried to follow.

At twelve-thirty, I wiped sweat from my forehead and pulled my shirt away from my chest. I felt like I was at a frat party. It felt good to dance, to let loose. We continued to move to the music until the band took a break. The sound level dropped, and a bar mix played over the speakers. Robyn turned and said she was going outside for a minute, but I didn't hear her. I was too preoccupied trying to catch my breath and cool down.

Without warning, she headed out of the bar. The moment I realized she was gone, I scrambled off the dance floor, walked through the crowded bar and headed out the front door in pursuit. I had lost sight of her and was worried she might have wanted to brush me off. Outside, I ran into her laughing with Holli and Lora. I was relieved she hadn't left before saying good night.

"It's getting late," I said, wondering how she would get home, but I didn't want to mess things up by being presumptuous. "Wanna crash at my place?" I cautiously asked. "No strings. We could walk down the hill and pick up your car in the morning?"

She hesitated, but finally answered, "Sounds good. If you don't mind, I probably shouldn't drive."

Robyn hugged Holli and Lora, and I turned and waved good-bye, as we headed down Main Street for the walk up the hill hand-in-hand.

When we arrived at my place, we walked into my apartment and bolted the door behind us. As I heard the lock click, I turned to Robyn, and our lips locked. As things heated up, my mind jumped to a question that I had nearly lost sight of. When was the right time to bring up the MS? I hadn't felt any symptoms since my body healed from the incident on the basketball court, but I didn't want to keep any secrets from her.

"Robyn there's something I need to tell you."

I stepped away from her and walked into the kitchen. Robyn walked to the opposite side of the kitchen counter and stood across from me. I watched her face switch from pleasure to concern.

"I have been diagnosed with multiple sclerosis."

Everything I had read about sharing health conditions said this was the wrong way to go about sharing my MS, but I wasn't operating on logic. I followed my heart, contrary to my usual guarded ways and shared the story of how I had been diagnosed four years earlier. I went on to tell her that I pushed myself physically and professionally to prove the disease didn't affect me, that it had led me to live a life bigger than I otherwise might have if I hadn't been diagnosed. I'm not sure she totally bought my rah-rah, glass-is-half-full talk, but it didn't matter, because she was ready to talk.

Robyn told me she had a family friend who had been diagnosed with MS when she was a kid. The last she heard was the woman required a cane to walk. I optimistically repeated what I had said about pushing myself physically and professionally, and that I hoped to keep the disease at bay. My secret sucked all of the passion out of the room. I walked around the counter and drew Robyn in for an extended embrace. I had a crazy strong connection with her and needed to hug her and feel like everything was going to be okay.

Rather than try to heat things back up, I asked if Robyn wanted to borrow a t-shirt and a pair of shorts to sleep in. She said yes, and we both got ready for bed. We got under the covers and went to sleep face-to-face, our noses three inches apart and woke up about the same way the next morning with the sun streaming into the room. I wasn't anxious or uneasy about her being there. It felt really good; like she was supposed to be with me.

We left my place holding hands and made our way down Hill Street to Robyn's Jeep. I guided my bike in my free hand, pleased to have these last few moments with her, wondering when we might see each other again. As we walked, she didn't ask about the MS, and I worried she had no interest in a second date.

When we arrived at the Jeep, I gave her a hug and kiss on the cheek. I wanted to kiss her on the lips but decided against it. Before I rode away, I suggested we get together the following weekend when I returned from Texas. My heart pounded; I couldn't resist asking her out. "I'd like to take you to dinner next Sunday night."

Robyn's face registered neither excitement nor surprise, leaving me with no true indication about how she really felt about the invitation.

"Sounds good. Why don't you give me a call from Texas, and we can talk about it," she said. That was Robyn. Naturally cooler than I could ever be. Sunday seemed like a lifetime from then, and by the time it arrived, my life would change again.

9

A MOMENT OF CLARITY AT COYOTE FLATS

What Robyn didn't know was that I was already in love—with mountains. The rugged solitude was a perfect environment for my troubled soul. Though I was excited to see her again, our date would happen at the end of my ultimate adventure weekend with Brendan: three days of mountain biking and climbing in the High Sierras. I hoped the trip would help me reach a new endurance threshold for my first triathlon in September. If I had any intimate relationship at the time, it was with my bike.

The approach to Coyote Flats began at 8,000 feet then ascended another 3,000 feet along a five-mile jeep trail. The grade was more than 14 % in stretches, on par with an unrated category climb in the Tour de France, except there would be no pavement. We had experience with steep climbs from our rides up the beasts around Southern California: Bulldog, Hell Hill, and E-Ticket. The challenge in the Sierra was the altitude and the rutted condition of the trail. I wasn't sure how I'd fare.

Ten minutes into the ride, it started to drizzle. Welcomed at first—the rain improved our traction—but two miles into the climb, a steady downpour soaked us. The cold numbed my hands and feet. Though the weather was less than ideal, the experience beat a morning behind a desk. We climbed well and pushed the pedals non-stop for more than an hour; neither of us dropped a foot to pause—a badge of honor on a tough climb.

Halfway up the hill, my body screamed for mercy. Just when I needed a break, we happened upon an abandoned shelter that resembled a bus stop, jutting out from the hillside. We took advantage of our good fortune and ducked inside for a short break to recharge. The hut was about fifteen feet by fifteen feet, with a leaky tin roof and trash strewn from end to end, but it shielded us from the rain and allowed us to rest before we got back on our bikes and climbed for another hour. Due to the cold, my fingers and toes had lost feeling. My legs ached and my lungs burned, but I stayed on Brendan's wheel. I wanted to show him that I was a worthy companion.

When we finally reached the summit at 11,000 feet, I struggled to breathe. I looked out across the barren, rocky terrain and felt like I was on the moon. We had crossed the tree line 1,000 feet below. After we crossed the summit, we bombed down a brief 800-foot descent and found ourselves at the base of the northern edge of Coyote Flats. Although we looked out on a beautiful highland meadow, we were 6,000 feet above the town of Bishop, in a highland valley that was crowned by 13,000-foot Sierra peaks.

We rode along the northern edge of the flats until we reached a fork in the road and a decision: go left and cruise back to Bishop for beers, or go right and head south across the flats—ten miles of the highly-anticipated cross-country fire road, then five miles of screaming downhill single track, and finally a nine-mile 'easy' cruise back to camp. We stopped and considered our decision over Pringles. I was wet and tired, so I welcomed the break. It was only eleven thirty, and we were making good time but we had worked too hard to choose the easy way out. We decided to stick to the plan.

Clouds had shrouded the peaks and walled us in as we continued across the flats. It was like we were in our own cloud cathedral. I looked out over the high mountain meadow and saw no signs of civilization other than the single-lane dirt road we followed. We encountered only two other people, a couple driving an SUV, as we rode. I secretly wanted to hop in the back seat and warm up, but there was no way I could surrender now.

At the southwestern end of the flats, we came to another intersection. The guidebook said to climb a mile to 10,290 feet, then descend to Baker Cabin. The clouds still enveloped us, but the rain had slowed to a spit. When we reached the top of the climb, my hands and feet felt like ice blocks. I was elated to see a cabin come into view, though it seemed like an aberration in the mist. We raced down the hill, hopped off our bikes, and went inside to investigate.

It was bare bones: a few chairs and a cot in one corner, but the real find was the potbelly stove in the middle of the room. Brendan, a former Eagle Scout, gave it the once-over. It checked out, so we rummaged around and gathered trash and debris to burn. Brendan found some matches, and after a few minutes, we had a roaring fire. We took off our shoes, socks, and shirts and put them on the stove to dry.

We sat next to the stove for an hour. As the fire blazed, we shared stories, laughed, and ate lunch. I spoke about my upcoming date with Robyn, and Brendan talked about the child he and his wife expected in a few months. The thought crossed my mind to tell Brendan about the MS, but I feared that if he knew, he might think twice about future trips. I could count on nine fingers the people who I'd told about the MS: Robyn, my parents, Pete, Aunt Sue, Uncle John, Matt, Terry, and Frank.

Telling Brendan didn't feel right. Everything had been perfect up until then, despite the inclement weather. We were going to tough it out no matter what. Rested, recharged, and warm, I was ready to finish the 5,000-foot single-track descent. I pulled my shirt off the stove to dress; it felt like I'd just pulled it from the dryer. We spread the coals, straightened up, and walked out of the cabin. I immediately noticed the rain had stopped, and the sun had broken through the clouds for the first time all day, and my optimism returned. We reviewed the plan one last time. We expected to arrive at our Baker Creek campsite by five o'clock, a two-and-a-half hour journey at most.

The path we took looked more like a seldom-used footpath than a maintained mountain bike trail, but since it was the only route, we assumed it was right and followed it. We headed downhill and walked the bikes around large rocks and branches—a clear indication we were off course, but we were too focused on our goal to notice.

We stopped at an overlook to take stock of our location. Brendan wanted to go northwest along the ridge. I made a case for southeast in the direction of the stream, the opposite way. I figured as long as we kept the creek in sight, we'd eventually end up back where we camped the night before. Brendan wanted more assurance.

I heard him unzip and rummage through his bag.

"Chando, I searched all the pockets and pouches in this thing, but I can't find it."

"Find what?"

"My compass."

I had a sinking feeling in my gut.

"Did you look in your repair kit? Maybe you stuffed it in there?"

"I looked, it's not there. I must have left it in the car at our campsite."

The one piece of gear guaranteed to help us finish the journey was warm and dry in his car. We approximated our position on the map and agreed to head east along Baker Creek. Though I wasn't sure we were going the right way, it felt good to head downhill. In my mind, we were making progress. We had taken action. We were in control.

Without a compass, hidden under the cover of trees and enveloped by fog that obscured all landmarks, we relied on the landscape immediately in front of us, trying our best to identify our location on the map. We would later learn we were forty-five degrees off course. We were supposed to travel due south, but instead we headed southeast into the trail-less, rugged backcountry of the Sierra without a compass or cell phone reception.

When we weren't bushwhacking, we picked our way downhill and bounded from one large rock to the next with twenty-pound bikes on our backs. After three hours, as the sun went down, the thought crossed my mind that we might be lost.

I wanted to find solace in the fact that we were scurrying along the bank of Baker Creek, where we had slept the previous night, but it was obvious we had missed the much-anticipated single-track trail we should have bombed down hours earlier. I assumed we just needed to put our heads down and bull through, and that eventually we'd return to camp. I conveniently looked past the 2000-foot mountain between us and the road. Denial was a familiar state, so alarm bells didn't sound—at least not yet.

By nine o'clock it was dark and my bike had grown heavy. I didn't have food or water to last beyond the trip we'd planned to end at five o'clock, four hours earlier. My race shoes worked well clipped to the pedals, but as I hiked downhill, my feet felt like they were strapped to woodblocks. I was tired and began to trip. At one point, I stumbled over a rock. One end of the handlebars jabbed me in the rib, and the other end struck me below the right eye. I sat to regroup. My rib ached and my eye stung, but I ignored the pain and tried to remain positive.

Surrounded by darkness, I dropped the bike where I stood, feeling the pain of leaving it up there. I had ridden my bike between fifty and seventy-five miles every week for the past two years, but I could no longer carry it.

I was convinced Brendan was a freak of nature because he still carried his bike. I however, moved better without mine and was encouraged for a few hundred feet, until we reached the impasse I'd hoped to avoid—a huge rock wall that rose a few hundred feet from the streambed, with no way to cross the water successfully without going over waterfalls. We finally realized we needed to climb the northwest ridge and began to scramble uphill to get around the wall and falls.

We climbed for two hours, until we finally reached the top of the ridge. We looked down and saw a steep face that led to the Owens Valley. That was *a* way to our camp, but not *the* way; it was too steep.

We decided to spend the night on the ridge with civilization in sight. We dug a hole with our hands. I crawled in and cuddled up to the rocks. Before I drifted off to sleep, I thought about seeing Robyn on our date Sunday, assuming I would return safely to Santa Monica. I saw us laughing about my experience over a bottle of wine. I imagined how much fun we'd have rehashing my war story. I just needed to persevere.

Brendan woke me from a dead sleep. When I opened my eyes, it was pitch black and I hoped I might be dreaming. "Chando," he called.

"I need to get moving," he said as his teeth chattered. "I'm freezing and I'm concerned about hypothermia. We need to move."

Brendan had early signs: intense shivering and cold pale skin. I groggily rose from the hole and brushed off my dirt blanket. This was no dream, it was a living nightmare. I was warmer than Brendan; he had given me his long-sleeve thermal shirt earlier in the night, even though we were both cold. When I asked him why seven years later, wondering if he suspected anything like MS, he said no, he gave me the shirt because he knew I needed it more.

We had been off-course for over ten hours. We were cold, tired, hungry, cut up, and my ribs were sore. We needed to climb 1,000 feet before we could turn east and descend another 2,000 feet of treacherous terrain before we got to the road. Before we pressed on guided by starlight, Brendan did something I would have never expected. He, too, left his bike. It was then that I realized our lives were in jeopardy.

After three hours of a slow uphill grind, I stopped to rest. I was moving better than Brendan, so I waited for him to catch up. I sat on a rock and stared ahead. I began to hallucinate. I saw something that terrified me—a black bear. They were known to inhabit this part of the Sierras, so I wasn't surprised, but I was scared. Should I run, or yell to Brendan for help? I sat paralyzed. If I ran, the bear would surely chase me, and he was probably a lot faster than me. Before I yelled for help, I took a closer look and realized the "bear" was just a tree stump. I laughed at myself, and my anxiety dissipated. Relieved, I waited for Brendan and looked toward the brightening horizon, believing we would escape our nightmare.

Brendan arrived at my rock a couple minutes later. I didn't tell him about my hallucination because I didn't want him to think I had lost my mind. He sat next to me and took out the map. We had gained enough ground, and it was time to head east. After we traveled for an hour, the ridge fell away and opened into a highland valley intersected by a road, the road we were supposed to cruise down on our bikes the previous afternoon.

Early Saturday morning, we hopped over a drainage ditch and stood on Glacier Lodge Road, too exhausted to celebrate. We staggered a hundred yards down the road in our helmets and bike shoes, hitchhiking. A truck pulled up and we told an abridged version of our story to the driver who dropped us at our campsite fifteen minutes later. We broke camp and splurged for a hotel in Bishop to clean up and get a few hours of desperately needed sleep. By one o-clock, after a shower and a nap, we felt human again.

We spent the next few hours stopping at search and rescue stations in Bishop, Independence and Lone Pine, hoping to hire a helicopter to find our bikes. None were available, rather they were being reserved for a 'real emergency.' Tired and demoralized, we headed back to LA We had lost our bikes but were happy to escape with our lives.

I met Robyn at the World Café Sunday night bearing a black eye and a three-inch bruise on my chest. Though I had slept well the night before, I felt beat up.

"Holy crap, what happened to you!" Robyn said when she saw me at the bar.

I looked down sheepishly. "It's a long story; let's take a seat in the lounge."

Robyn examined my arms and pulled up my pant legs seeing gashes, scrapes, and bruises. "Ouch! Tell me all about it."

"The trip didn't exactly go as planned."

"That's obvious," she said.

I told her the trip was magical up to the point when we left the cabin and started out across the back country.

"You had the bikes the whole time?"

"No, I left mine in a canyon at about nine that night after I tripped and fell. That's when I got the black eye. Brendan left his by the hole we slept in."

"That's crazy. I had a dream Friday night that you had a black eye."

"Wild. We must have some crazy cosmic connection," I said.

She paused and smiled. "Maybe so."

10

FACING TERROR IN TEXAS

Robyn and I dated three months and had become a couple. I started to miss her more and more each time I boarded the plane for Houston. I was surprised she had such a huge effect on me. After I landed and drove to Huntsville to begin my week of work, I would call her to chat, knowing she had Mondays off.

During one such conversation, I worked up the courage to ask her about how she felt about moving in together. I knew it was soon, but I also knew we had something special. I wanted to get a feel for where I stood. It was the first time I had ever broached the topic with any woman I had dated. I knew we had only been together for a few months, so I chose my words carefully. I didn't want to scare her.

Robyn wasn't at all interested in my suggestion of co-habitation. She was raised to be independent and had supported herself for the previous twelve years. She had lived with a guy in her early twenties and taken on the responsibilities of a wife. She adapted her personality to fit what she thought the guy wanted. The relationship jaded her perspective on men and led her to believe that she wouldn't get married and would probably have to raise a child on her own. She didn't need a roommate, and she certainly wasn't looking for a marriage proposal. She wanted someone to love her for the real her. I would learn she had just ended a two-year relationship and was surprised to find herself in another so suddenly.

I was equally surprised by our relationship. I had planned to spend the summer traveling back and forth to Texas and training for the Malibu triathlon, while she intended to spend the summer partying like a rock star before her 30th birthday that fall. As we talked, I realized our budding courtship probably would have been suffocating had we not been apart Monday through Thursday. I realized I would have to take things slow.

Still, I wanted to be closer to her. The thought of leaving the Texas project had crossed my mind, but I didn't give it serious consideration. Ever since my days of high school basketball, quitting wasn't an option. In tenth grade, I had made the boys' junior varsity basketball team. I wanted to be a power forward, but I wasn't big enough. The first time I realized my height limitations was during a mid-season game, in which I hadn't played a minute. I rode home with my parents after the game and pouted in the back seat, insisting I was going to quit. My dad challenged me.

"You know, Jon, I can understand how you feel, but I'm not sure quitting is the answer. There were probably a dozen guys who were cut and another dozen who thought about trying out but didn't. Aren't you grateful you made the team?"

"I guess so."

"If you quit, you will let all of your buddies down. You don't want to be known as a quitter, do you?"

"No . . . ," I said, with a hint of fifteen-year-old attitude.

I felt like that pouty kid again. I hated that I had to work long, windowless hours separated from Robyn. Her growing importance in my life caused me to question my commitment to the project, but I let the feeling pass—our relationship was young and there was no guarantee we'd stay together, so I decided against quitting early, if ever.

♦

The second week of September, I followed my usual Monday routine and flew to Texas in the morning and arrived at the office after lunch. I moved through the rest of my day intently focused. I wanted to leave by eight o'clock, so I could eat dinner and get to the high school track for my evening run. Training was the only thing that kept me motivated during the long days in Texas. As I left the office, I felt confident that I had nailed the next day's performance review.

A guy was coming in town from the D.C. office to put me through my paces and make sure the plan I had developed for the next project phase was sound. I drove away from the office relieved to see nothing but acres of green pastures on my way to the track. I could see the amber glow of the late-summer sunset from my rearview mirror, thinking Huntsville was an idyllic rural community.

The thought vaporized the instant I drove past the guard towers and twelve-foot razor wire that rimmed the chain link fences of the Byrd Unit, a maximum-security prison. By the time I reached the parking lot in front of the track, the sun had set, and I was spooked. Instead of conveying a sense of security, the guard towers and fences made me anxious. What if a prisoner escaped and grabbed me and took me hostage while I ran?

I parked and walked to the infield to stretch. I was relieved to see four lights at each turn along the track. I found a place to sit in the cool moist grass and loosened up, not just from sitting at the office, but from all the time I'd spent cramped on a plane. I stretched my legs and lined up at the track's midpoint, hearing the evening's first crickets.

I reset my stopwatch, pushed start, and was off. I ran at a good pace and counted each deep breath to focus my mind. After I had completed about a third of a lap, I had counted twenty breaths and checked my watch; it read thirty seconds. I hit my stride in the straightaway and felt like I was flying. I yearned for my body to remember this rush, unsure how long the MS would allow me the luxury of this harmony. I pushed my body to run all-out for 400 meters, finished the lap, and walked back to the starting line and did it eleven more times, completing each lap in about eighty seconds.

At that pace, I could possibly run four laps (a mile) in under six minutes. If I could do that twenty-six times, I would be able to run a two-hour-and-forty-minute marathon. That was a pipe dream, so I factored in a 25% decline in performance to account for recovery. Still, I could qualify for the Boston Marathon. Something beyond my goal was working to keep me on the track each night in Texas. In the back of my mind, I thought that if I ran fast enough, someday, I might even outrun the MS. The next morning on September 11, I arrived at the office first thing and met with Jim for the daylong progress review. After two hours, we took a break, and I walked into the team area. A somber mood hung over the office. Something was up. I walked to Garrett's desk to see what was happening.

"What's up? A lot of the team isn't here, and those who are have their heads down," I said.

"We're under attack."

"What do you mean, attack?" as if I didn't understand the meaning of the word. Garrett wasn't one for drama. He was a straight shooter, and I liked that about him.

"Well, Chando," Garrett said in his authoritarian Texan drawl used to tell tales of shooting eight-point bucks in Hill Country with his buddies, "It's all over the news."

"What's all over the news?"

"The Twin Towers were hit by two passenger jets and are no longer standing; the Pentagon was hit by a third plane and is on fire, and a fourth plane crashed in a field in Pennsylvania."

"*What the fuck?*" I said. I was overcome by a tremendous sense of sorrow that quickly turned to fear. I stood there silent and motionless, trying to make sense of what I had heard. I don't remember what I said to Garrett next. I only remember what I did—I turned around and went back to work. I had a project review to pass and a job to do. This was the only way I knew how to deal with something bigger than I could handle. If I didn't acknowledge the tragedy, I didn't have to feel much of anything—just like the MS. After returning to the conference room and agreeing to take a break with Jim, I walked out of the office and through the mall to a café. The gravity of the news hadn't settled. I placed my order and looked at my watch. It was a little after eight o'clock on the West Coast. Robyn might still be asleep, but would be getting up soon for work. I took a chance waking her.

"Morning babe," I said when she answered.

"Hey, so good to hear your voice."

It sounded like she had been awake for a while.

"You're up early," I said.

"Holli called first thing. Her mom in Massachusetts called to tell her the news and make sure she was okay and then she called me. I turned on the TV in time to see the second tower go down. I didn't think it was real. It was like some kind of bizarre movie. I sat for a while in front of the TV in shock and cried. It was so scary!"

Robyn's dad had served as a cop for thirty years, and the news hit hard. For the first time in our relationship, I heard terror as she recounted the events. I wanted to be at Robyn's side, rather than eighteen hundred miles and a four-hour plane ride away. I felt the loneliness of the expanse, but there was no time to deal with those feelings. We hung up and agreed to talk later.

I ate my breakfast and walked back into the conference room and waited for Jim.

"Alright Chando, let's get through this. I'll probably try to get back home this afternoon, so let's move through the rest of your slides and wrap up before lunch, then get a pulse on things."

Jim and I were very focused for the next two hours. We moved through my material and broke for lunch, when I walked into the team area and found Garrett.

"Chando, you heard? The President has closed the airspace over the U.S. until further notice. No planes are flying."

My mind raced. Our country was being attacked. The world was facing Armageddon and I was two thousand miles from Robyn. How would I get to her?

Then it came to me—drive. It would be a long trip. I had never driven that distance in one stretch, but I figured if I drove through the night and drank enough caffeine, I could be in LA the following evening. I went to find Jim and shared my plan to get home to Robyn. The news from New York trumped anything on our desks.

He agreed. "I'm going to drive my rental car up to DC to be with my wife."

I hopped in my car, dropped by my apartment, packed a few things, and hit the road. I called Robyn to let her know. "I'm coming home," I said when she answered.

"What!? How are you going to get here? No planes are flying," she said.

"I'm going to drive."

"You're crazy! Isn't that like a thousand miles?"

"It's one thousand seven hundred and eighty miles."

"So, I'll see you when . . . Saturday?"

"Nope. I'll see you by the time you get home from work tomorrow night."

"I don't know if that's such a good idea," she said.

"I'm packed and already on the road. I'll be home tomorrow afternoon," I said determined to drive 80 miles per hour through the night.

I wasn't sure what to expect with the world crashing down around me. I was surprised that the highways were clear, and I made good time through Texas. Just after midnight, I crossed the Texas/New Mexico border. I was having a hard time keeping my eyes open, so I exited the highway and checked into a hotel.

Before I went to sleep, I called Robyn to give her an update. It was eleven o'clock on the West Coast and she was still awake. I let her know I had pulled over to get some sleep.

The next morning, as I drove through Southern New Mexico, the sun sat high in the sky. The deep blue was punctured by puffy white clouds, and many rocky buttes and mesas that rose out of the desert. The setting provided plenty of space to think, and it became clear that being with Robyn was all that mattered.

I finally entered Los Angeles at twilight. As I turned off Interstate 10 and onto National Boulevard, a rush of adrenalin pulsed through my haggard body. I was only a few minutes from holding Robyn. I pulled into an empty space in front of her building and rushed through the front door and up the elevator to her apartment.

I must have looked terrible. I had just driven eighteen hundred miles in a day and a half. I was strung out on caffeine, and my eyes felt like sandpaper had rubbed them, but when I knocked and Robyn opened the door, I knew I was home and safe in her embrace.

11

A SWEET RELEASE

The events of the previous week had caused me to reevaluate my priorities. My relationship with Robyn had become much more important. I had no way of knowing how this reordering of things would impact my relationship with MS, or if it would have any impact at all. Would I be able to live in denial and still find harmony with Robyn?

I followed through with my triathlon commitment and completed the race at the end of September. During the fall, I flew back and forth to LA on weekends to be with Robyn. Though I was in Texas during the week, I tried to make her a bigger part of my life. I asked her to fly to Philadelphia to meet my family over Thanksgiving and watch me run the marathon. She took a red-eye from California to watch Pete and me run past the Philadelphia Zoo at mile eight.

As Pete and I ran in stride, I stared ahead toward the zoo entrance and spotted Robyn's red sweater and black coat next to my parents. When I reached her, I stopped, gave her a big hug, and told her how happy I was to see her.

"It's so good to see you; we just got here. I have some funny stories to tell you about getting here," she said, gesturing toward my father.

I turned and hugged my mom and gave my father a high five, then no sooner did Pete and I get back in stride did I turn around and sprint back to Robyn. I wanted her to know how much I appreciated the effort she made to fly out and see me.

"I'm so happy that you're here." I said then hugged her and ran back to Pete.

"I can't wait to see you at the finish," she yelled back.

At mile twenty-three, my muscles screamed for mercy. My paced had slowed considerably since I'd seen Robyn, and my goal of finishing in three hours and thirty minutes was in jeopardy. I looked over at Pete, who seemed to be running effortlessly.

"Pete, why don't you run ahead? My muscles ache, and I need to slow down."

"I'm not going anywhere; I told you I looked forward to crossing the finish-line next to you. If you need to walk, then we walk."

"But I don't want to slow you down," I pleaded.

"Jon, I don't care about my time, I want to cross the finish line together."

I looked down at my watch. We had been running for three hours and thirty minutes. I realized qualifying for Boston wasn't possible and turned my focus to a new goal—to finish under four hours. I had about thirty minutes to run the last two miles. I was bummed about Boston but was pleased to still have a shot at finishing with a respectable time. Just then Jay, my best friend from high school, appeared.

"Johnny boy, I'm here to run you and Pete to the finish," he said as he ran onto the course. I was surprised to see him; we hadn't discussed him running with us to the finish. But that was Jay, always there to support a friend. I had been running on fumes and received a kick of energy seeing him. Having him at my side to run the last two miles was a blessing. At mile twenty-six, I heard Robyn's screams of encouragement.

"Come on Jon, you can do it, just a little bit further, you're doing great!"

Hearing Robyn's cheering, I ran the last four hundred feet at the best sprint I could muster and crossed the finish line with Jay and Pete at my side. I looked up at the clock: three hours and fifty-five minutes. I finished in under four hours. I stopped to hug Pete and Jay. "Thanks for getting me across the line. If it wasn't for you guys, I would still be back at mile twenty-four asking myself why I was doing this."

I made my way through finishers, looking to find Robyn and my parents. Robyn greeted me with another big hug.

"Congratulations! You did such a great job!"

What she didn't tell me was that she was very concerned and had expected me at the finish at the three-hour-and-thirty-minute mark—the time I told her I hoped to finish and qualify for Boston. She had been worrying about my welfare for the previous twenty-five minutes. I was groggy and my response to questions was delayed another cause for her worry. I was so overheated, it was affecting my eyesight, and she could tell. She hid her concern while we took pictures and celebrated, while I denied that anything was wrong; I assumed my body's 'slurring' was just the result of completing a marathon.

As Robyn, Pete and I drove home, I asked her how it went meeting my parents at the airport. "Did you recognize them?"

"They were standing at the bottom of the escalator as I went to baggage claim and greeted me with big warm smiles. I recognized them from pictures. After the airport, your dad drove me all over town looking for coffee."

"There isn't much between the airport and South Philly."

"No there wasn't, but your father was on a mission."

"Dad's like a dog with a bone when you tell him you need something."

Robyn smiled and nodded, playing along with our charade. Without saying a word or even shaking a hand, she had signed the covenant of keeping my family's secrets.

The day after Thanksgiving, I put Robyn on a flight to Los Angeles so that she could get back to work. Our week in Philadelphia was all I had hoped it would be. Robyn mixed well with my family and friends. She made a great impression on everyone.

On Sunday afternoon, I boarded a flight back to Houston and thought about our relationship. It was clear: she was my soul mate. I just needed to figure out a way to get off the prison project and get back to Santa Monica, so that we could be in the same city and confirm that our relationship worked day-to-day, not just weekend-to-weekend.

We had spent every weekend together the previous seven months, but our relationship felt like a string of third dates. We were both on our best behavior because we knew our time together was limited. We didn't take on the hard issues. We avoided MS, but there was no doubt it was the pink elephant in the room that we both ignored.

Robyn had noticed a few things about my condition in the time we had been dating. I had a delayed reaction when I was stressed and squinted when I was overheated. She let her concerns go because we had only been dating for seven months. Our relationship remained in a holding pattern for the next five months; I flew into LA on Fridays and flew back to Houston on Monday mornings twenty-three times. In April of 2002, the project moved out of the implementation phase and into the testing phase. I knew these transitions offered the perfect chance to reconfigure teams, and it was time to reconfigure the relationship I had with Robyn.

I saw my opportunity to leave the project. We had regained the confidence of the Texas Department of Criminal Justice, and there was a young guy brought onto the team a few months earlier with the skills to take over my responsibilities. I scheduled a meeting with the manager of day-to-day project delivery so I could ask to be rolled off the project. I sat down with him at our scheduled time and got right to it.

"I have someone special back in Santa Monica, who I think is the one, but who I've only dated since being on the project. I need to get back to Santa Monica to be sure."

"Are you asking to be taken off the project?"

"I am."

"Well, I appreciate all you've done to help get us back on track. I'm sorry you won't be here to see us take the application live."

"Me, too."

"I'll talk with the account executive and see when it makes sense to roll you off."

"Thanks, please make it as soon as possible."

"Do you have a project to go back to when you return?"

"I don't."

"I'll see what I can do to make it happen by the end of the month."

So I was off the project? Just like that? I rose from the table and returned to the team area, incredulous, knowing our conversation had lasted only fifteen minutes. I had put myself through hell over the previous twelve months, flying more than 100,000 miles during my time in Texas, only to realize that to stop the chaos, all I needed to do was ask.

12

FIGURE IT OUT

My first Saturday back in LA, Robyn and I spent a romantic weekend in the heart of Santa Ynez Valley Wine Country to reconnect and celebrate our first year anniversary as a couple, but it didn't turn out the way either of us wanted. Robyn was very loving and open, but I was standoffish and emotionally unavailable. She tried numerous times to get me to open up. She talked about how excited she was for me to be back in Santa Monica so we could spend more time together, but getting me to talk about how I felt was like pulling teeth. The harder she tried the more I resisted.

I took the following week off from work as comp time for my fourteen months of service in Texas, and I spent the week hiking and riding by myself to try and work through my feelings. The outcome of my brooding was vague. I was no clearer about what I really wanted with Robyn than at the start of the week. If anything, I was more confused. I didn't have the emotional skills to let my feelings guide me into any decision.

We spent Friday night together, and the following Saturday morning, we dressed and hopped in Robyn's Jeep so she could drop me at my place on her way to work. It felt like miles separated us inside the

Jeep, and I looked out the window, feeling awkward. That's when Robyn brought up a subject I had successfully avoided for the previous year.

"What are you going to do about the MS?"

"What do you mean? I'm going to run and ride my bike and keep the diagnosis from impacting my life," I said, the words sounding rehearsed.

"That's not what I mean. I'm amazed with all you do to stay in shape, but I think it would be good to develop a relationship with an MS specialist to make sure you do everything possible to remain unaffected."

I stared out the window and watched her accelerate past traffic. This was the last thing I wanted to talk about.

"You know, there isn't a cure for MS," I said. "The only thing you can do is take a drug to maybe delay its onset. I don't even know whether the disease will ever impact me. I'm doing a pretty good job without taking any of the drugs and don't think I need a doctor."

"I hope that continues to be the case, but if we're going to stay together and have a future, I need to know you are doing everything you can to keep the MS in check."

I sat in silence. Robyn had never given me an ultimatum before, and I needed to sit with it before I responded.

The following week, I used my second week of comp time to hike up White Mountain, another California 14er, and sort things out. As I climbed, I considered what I liked about Robyn. I was attracted to her strong free spirit and her fearlessness, how she moved to California to forge her own identity. I liked that she always remained positive in the face of challenges. If we shared a life together and I did become impacted by the diagnosis, Robyn seemed to possess the right mindset to weather hard times.

I also liked that Robyn worked hard. We had both spent significant parts of our childhoods in New England and shared a Puritan work ethic. She stood on her feet eight hours per day, six days per week.

Robyn also had a strong sense of family. Her parents were married for more than thirty years, so she had watched them deal with the ups and downs of life. She was also close with her only sibling, her sister Raylene, and wanted to have children. And while her blond-haired, blue-eyed beauty never escaped me, what struck me most was her resolve to live honestly. She made decisions based on her instincts, and I admired her integrity. I was pleased our values aligned but her desire to get married remained an open question along with her desire for me to face the MS if we decided to stay together.

I reached the summit and took a seat. I looked out over the Owens Valley nine thousand feet below and saw the snow-capped Sierra Mountains off in the distance. As I gazed at the dramatic beauty, I started to think hard about our compatibility. Hiking back to the Jeep, I thought about how easily Robyn expressed her emotions, but I wondered how I could ever match her emotional honesty and literacy. It wouldn't be fair if Robyn kept giving and got nothing in return. What also concerned me was Robyn's penchant for perfection. I was a perfectionist, too, and didn't know if I could meet *her* expectations. The most pressing question was whether or not I was ready to face the MS. I still needed more time to answer that, and I returned from my hike confused. I was a skilled project manager, but managing the MS was not something I felt even remotely capable of doing. It was easier to work sixty hours a week than face the work I needed to do on myself.

I had the rest of the week off from work and rode my bike fiercely, trying to summon the courage to talk to Robyn. Sunday came and I still hadn't found what I needed to know or say. We sat together on her couch and discussed the week ahead.

"Robyn, There's something I need to talk about."

She stared at me, surprised. I never called her by her first name. I said 'Babe' almost every time I addressed her. She knew I had something important to say, already in tune with my near radio silence since I had returned from Texas.

"What's up?"

"I've thought a lot about our relationship."

"I'm listening," she said.

"Now that I'm back from Texas, I need some time to myself."

"So, what you're saying is that you are breaking up with me?"

I sat, processing the gravity of the words, and my eyes welled up.

"I need some time to myself, to make sure I'm ready to spend more time together."

I didn't have the courage to tell her the real reason was because I was too afraid to face the MS.

"Don't wait too long," Robyn shot back. "I may not be waiting."

I couldn't get out of her place fast enough. I hopped off the couch and jumped in my Jeep. My mind raced about what I had just done. I felt tremendous sorrow. I had tightness in my chest and struggled to catch my breath. What had I done? I returned from Texas to spend time with Robyn, but rather than come closer, I'd run away.

I was scared to love someone. I remembered a conversation I had with my Uncle John in the den of his home in Marblehead just after I completed the LA Marathon. We sat watching a Red Sox game, and he asked, "Jon, why do you run?"

"I love the feeling," I said.

I realized what my uncle was really asking that day was, "What are you running from?" I didn't know it then, but I was running *in order to feel*. It was my way to feel pain, and in that way, to connect with myself. I would come to realize the slow paralysis, almost always associated as a symptom of MS, was partly the consequence of denying my emotions for most of my life. But that was a lesson for another day.

I got home and looked for things to do to distract me. I paid my bills and thought about the week ahead. On Monday, I was grateful to have a lot on my plate at work, so I didn't have time to think about Robyn.

On Wednesday after work, I returned home and put on my running shoes for an eight-mile run by the ocean. I needed to think and really needed to feel. I had no idea how I'd spend the weekend without Robyn. I ran the last two miles fast. I reached my apartment gasping for air and felt a pinch in my side. I was used to runner's cramps, but this wasn't one. It was the pain of not being with Robyn.

I arrived at work on Thursday morning and read through my email. When I finished reading my last message, I sent her an email. I sent her a link to my favorite web video, "The Power of One," a source of inspiration and strength for me. I clicked the send button and waited for her response. Within two hours she replied: Indigo Girls, *Swamp Ophelia*, track 5, "The Power of Two."

"Touché," I replied back.

The next day I left the office at 5:00. When I got home, I gave into my urge and picked up the phone and called Robyn.

"What's up?" she asked.

"I thought maybe we could get together on Saturday night and talk. I miss you."

"Actually, I have plans." There was an awkward silence on the line. It felt like I had received a stiff kick. Had she found someone else? Her comment threw me into more of a tailspin than the morning I received the results of my first MRI. I tried to compose myself, and she didn't torture me any longer. "But I'm available on Sunday."

I took a deep breath.

"How about I bring a movie over?" I offered.

 "Sure. Why don't you come over at five."

"Sounds great!"

I hung up and jumped around my apartment. I didn't know it at the time, but she had the exact same reaction. I knew we had a lot to discuss before we reestablished our connection, but I was ecstatic to have a date set to see her.

Five o'clock on Sunday couldn't come fast enough. On the drive to Robyn's, I replayed a dozen times what I would say. I arrived at her door and knocked, rather than simply enter as I had done when we were together.

She opened the door and curtly said, "Come in."

I wanted to greet her with a big hug after our separation, but I felt it would have been presumptuous, so I didn't. I made my way to the couch. Robyn usually poured me a glass of red wine, but instead she took the seat next to me and quietly waited for me to make the next move. It was like our first date.

"How have you been?" I asked.

"Okay. How about you?"

 "I miss you."

"Well, you made the decision for us not to be together."

"I'm seriously questioning that."

"Oh yeah? Tell me."

I sat on the couch and groveled for her forgiveness. I told her what a jerk I had been and searched for the right words to show how remorseful I was, how important she was to me, and how much I wanted us to be back together. She finally ended my torture and said, "I forgive you, but you really hurt me, and it will take me some time to get over it."

I told her I understood and apologized again, hoping I could win her back.

13

LOOKING INTO THE MIRROR

Now that Robyn and I were in the same town, I was finally ready to confront my diagnosis—if anything to further develop our relationship. I spent most of my time at Robyn's place. I was busy at work but tried to keep a healthy balance.

One fall Sunday afternoon, during halftime of the Philadelphia Eagles football game, I ran to a neighborhood convenience store to pick up a soda and a bag of chips. I returned to watch the game and enjoy my snack. The moment I sat on the couch, Robyn said, "Those look good. Did you pick me up some popcorn?"

I sat, awestruck. "I didn't know you were hungry. If I'd known, I would have picked you up a bag."

"Did you ask?"

"Well, no . . . I was in a hurry to get a snack before the start of the second half, so I just ran down to the corner store."

"I'm not really hungry, but the next time you go on a snack run, you might want to ask if I want something, too."

"You were downstairs when I left, or I would have asked."

"Jon, you know you could have waited two minutes for me to put the laundry in the dryer, that included your dirty socks," Robyn shot back.

It made me angry to be challenged like that, but I liked how Robyn allowed me to see my shortcomings. "You're right, I should have."

After the game, Robyn joined me on the couch to watch a movie. It felt good to be next to her without having the nagging need to pack and fly to Houston.

She turned to me, broaching a familiar topic.

"Have you thought any more about an MS doctor?"

This time I didn't resist the conversation. I told her about the doctor I had seen three years ago, who was in East LA. I told her I wasn't sure how to find a Westside doctor, and said I didn't have time to search for one during my busy week ahead.

Robyn wouldn't let me slide. "You need to put your health, and more specifically the MS, higher on your priority list."

"Staying healthy is my highest priority," I said defiantly.

"Your actions need to show it. You want to run on the beach with your child someday, right?"

This was the first time we had discussed kids, and I became defensive. "Of course I do. There's no way the MS will prevent that from happening," I said.

"You need to ensure that happens by making sure you remain minimally impacted. I think having a doctor will help."

The conversation was like pulling teeth, but Robyn kept me honest. That week, she even did my homework for me. She came home with the name of a doctor. One of her clients was an MRI radiologist who read the films of MS patients and dealt with numerous neurologists in the area. He provided her with the name of a good one, Andy Woo, from Santa Monica Neurological Consultants.

When I saw Andy for the first time, we connected like no other doctor I had ever seen. He was a few years older than me. We both went to school back East and were avid Lakers fans. Andy took his first read on my condition. He put me through a battery of tests to examine my balance, cognitive, visual and audible acuity, as well as my strength and dexterity. He concluded I was minimally impacted. I knew that was the case, but it was nice to hear. Before we finished, Andy tried to convince me to take one of the MS therapies. He said I was in the A plus group of people who lived with MS and that taking one of the drugs was great insurance to make sure I remained minimally impacted.

Since the diagnosis five years earlier, I had stayed up on significant MS advancements. I knew there were new therapies available Avonex, Copaxone and Rebif, but I didn't consider any of them because I knew they were fundamentally the same as Betaseron. The Treatment my neurologist recommended I take when first diagnosed. They reduced the frequency of attacks by about a third, but none were a cure. And they each required an injection a few times a week if not every day which seemed like a lot of effort for minimal benefit, so I hadn't pursued them.

I told Andy I was aware of the four therapies—the CRAB drugs, as they were commonly referred: Copaxone, Rebif, Avonex, and Betaseron. I told him that since I had lived with the disease for several years, I wasn't ready to inject myself weekly, or even daily, but he made one final attempt to sway me.

"I hear what you're saying, but keep in mind that I want you to be minimally impacted, like the sixty- and seventy-year-old blue-haired women that come to see me. You can't tell they live with the disease."

At first, I wasn't sure why Andy's reference only included women, and then I remembered that three quarters of those affected by MS are women. Andy and I discussed the meaning of "minimally impacted." It meant these women walked into his office with no visible symptoms. I thought about those older patients and realized they might have been in their early thirties like me when they were diagnosed; they wouldn't have had the option of taking any of the current therapies because they hadn't been created, and these women still managed their MS fine. Andy's comment probably didn't have the intended effect. It actually comforted me and made me feel okay about not taking any medication. The disease hadn't yet forced my hand; I wasn't ready to lay down another bike.

♦

That fall, Pete and I ran the Philadelphia marathon over Thanksgiving for a second time. Robyn flew to watch me race and celebrate the holiday with my family. My body was in good condition, but my performance didn't compare to the previous year. I finished in four hours and twenty minutes, one-minute-per-mile slower.

I knew enough that my training had nothing to do with my lapsing time. At the mile-four water stop, I tangled legs with another runner, tripped and fell hard on my right elbow. I remember lying in a puddle of water on the pavement and watching the legs of upright, able-bodied runners pass. At first I feared I was having an MS attack and would need to drop out of the race. Pete, wrought with worry, rushed over to see if I was okay.

I looked at him and couldn't help but think of our walk on Crane's Beach the week I received the diagnosis—the day I had told him about my aspirations to live a great life. I probably had run more than 3,000 miles during the previous three years and never once tripped. Every second I lay on the cold, hard pavement counted against my finish time. I recalled the conversation with my Uncle John while I watched the other runners pass, and I realized for the first time that it didn't matter how fast I ran, because I might not ever be able to outrun MS.

I snapped out of it and answered Pete.

"My elbow hurts, but I think I'm okay. Let's keep going."

That was that. I gave no space for any more emotions. After a hundred yards, I could tell I was okay—not like the day on the basketball court. I had no hesitation or tightness in my legs, but I continued to think about my fall for the next twenty-two miles.

I desperately tried to jam my fear in the box of denial, but I couldn't stop my rational mind from drawing conclusions. I had tangled legs and tripped because MS had most likely impacted my ability to judge distance. At the finish line, I could hear Robyn's screams of encouragement.

"Come on Jon, you can do it, you're almost there; just a little further! COME ON, YOU CAN DO IT!"

When I crossed the finish line, I didn't have to fight my way through the crowd and search for Robyn like the year before. She ran up and hugged me.

"I'm so happy to see you," she said, full of relief. "What happened? Your parents and I expected you thirty-five minutes ago, the time you said you hoped to finish. When you weren't here at the four-hour mark, we started to panic, and I ran back down the course to look for you. I spotted you and Pete about a mile from the finish and ran along the sidelines cheering you on."

I looked into her eyes and saw the worry. I hadn't heard her cheering me on over the last mile and wasn't sure how to respond.

"I struggled this year. I tangled legs with another runner at the mile-four water stop and tripped. I landed hard on my right elbow. It's still sore," I said and raised my arm to show her the two-inch gash.

"Ouch, that looks like it hurts. Let me go and see if I can get you some ice."

"Where?"

"There's got to be some at the first aid station. I'll be right back."

I looked to my right, and Pete was standing there.

"How are you doing?" he asked, still worried.

"Okay. I'm tired and my elbow is sore, but we finished."

What I didn't tell him was that I was wiped out. I was overheated, my body ached, and my eyesight was a little blurry, but I didn't continue because my parents walked up. I hugged them and took a big breath, then let out a sigh of relief.

"Four hours and twenty-two minutes," my dad said.

"Yeah, it feels good to be finished."

His comment begged the question of how I felt and why I had finished over a minute-per-mile slower than last year, but I refused to go there. Robyn arrived with ice.

"Here you go, put this on your elbow."

"What happened?" my mom asked, startled.

"I tangled legs in a crowd of runners at the first water stop. You know how crowded things get at water stops. It bothered me the rest of the run," I said.

Pete, Robyn, and I separated from my parents and walked back to the car. Before we got in to drive home, Robyn took me aside.

"Jon, I was sick with worry as I ran back to look for you. I can't take any more. I don't want you to run marathons. Running a few miles is fine, but no more of this bullshit where you push yourself so hard; you might end up really hurting yourself. You just don't know when to stop."

Her words were hard to take. I knew I had pushed myself way past my limit to prove I could outrun the MS, and I knew better than to argue with her. My elbow bothered me for the next few months, but not any more than the fear of awakening MS from a deep sleep. That bear I had "seen" up on Coyote Flat was perhaps real and lurking.

Over the holidays, Robyn and I moved closer to a formal engagement. That Christmas, I gave her diamond earrings to show her my commitment. And as our bond grew deeper, MS became a more frequent topic of discussion. At the start of the year, I had the first of two biannual appointments with Andy. This time Robyn joined me. She sat in the chair next to me while Andy put me through the usual battery of tests.

"Jon, let's start with the films." Andy projected the eleven-by-seventeen-inch transparent images of my brain on the illuminated wall in front of his desk. "They look pretty clean. There are one or two new spots, and a couple of the preexisting spots are getting a little lighter; this indicates slight progression, but overall they look pretty good."

Spots were lesions on my brain where the myelin had worn away due to immune system attacks on my nervous system. Healthy brain matter looked dark gray and solid on film, while attacked brain matter was light gray.

"That doesn't sound too bad. What else do you see?" I asked.

"From the films and the results of your exam today, I'd still put you in the A plus category of people living with MS."

"That's good, right?" I asked.

"It is . . . ," he said uncertainly, as if to say, *That's one way to look at it.*

I denied the possibility of anything less than a positive outlook on my condition, but Robyn had a more realistic reaction to the news. She had seen the changes in my condition. All she could think was, "Preexsiting spots . . . slight progression . . . Oh shit!" Nothing about that sounded good, and it freaked her out, but she bit her tongue. All she really wanted to know was, *"How the fuck do we stop it?"*

Robyn and I wanted to do all we could to make sure I was minimally impacted as we moved closer to marriage. I knew how fortunate I was to be unaffected after living with the disease for six years, but the time lying in the puddle during the marathon made me wonder how much longer I could remain in the A plus group.

"Andy, what drug should I be taking?"

"You want to be minimally impacted, right?"

"Yes, I want to walk in here in my seventies like those blue-haired women."

"Rebif seems to be the most effective, if you can tolerate it."

"What does tolerate it mean?"

"As with any treatment, there are side effects. Rebif is a beta-interferon. It mimics the immune system and acts as a decoy to distract an overactive system from attacking myelin. Side effects include fatigue, weakness, and back pain."

The side effects didn't seem all that bad relative to the onset of symptoms. I could take the drug. I was no longer living my life alone, and I could see from Robyn's reaction that she wanted me to take it. I was anxious to please her but had one lingering objection.

"The Rebif needs to be injected, right?" I asked.

"Yes, three times a week."

"I'll help with injections," Robyn volunteered.

I looked at her lovingly and asked Andy to get the paperwork going. Robyn and I stood and walked out of the examination room. I kissed her on the back of the head.

"Does that feel better?" I asked.

She smiled.

That spring, we went through our lives like a young couple in love. We were on autopilot: we worked hard, enjoyed our time together, and I began to take the Rebif. Robyn brought out the best in me, and I was eager to formalize our commitment, so in April I began to shop for the perfect engagement ring and made reservations for our engagement weekend at Bacara Resort in mid-June to surprise her.

At the same time, I was planning to climb Mount Shasta the first weekend in June with Matt, my good buddy from MIT, two of his friends, Pete, and our friend Holly, who I had known from our days at the University of Richmond. These were the people who I wanted to sit with on the top of the world and celebrate my pending engagement.

14

DISCOVERING THE OUTER LIMITS

I knew that Shasta was a powerful mountain. The town nestled at her base attracts all sorts of characters—most seeking a combination of healing, clarity, metaphysical energy, and exhilaration. In all her glory, Shasta is a sleeping giant. You don't just visit her on a whim without preparing for the consequences of waking her, or her you. If she senses a climber needs awakening, she is poised to shake you out of your slumber.

I was ready for the challenge, conscious or not. I had climbed the mountain the year before with Brendan. I knew what to expect, and I had fully recovered from the Philadelphia marathon six months earlier; it was a distant memory. Things seemed perfect the Saturday morning when we started the climb up Avalanche Gulch. Blue skies. Fair weather. Zero wind. Snow just hard enough to walk across without sinking.

I thought I was prepared. I poured myself into the planning and managed the project as if Shasta was a client. I assembled the climbing team, arranged flights, coordinated equipment, and offered moral support to all invited. I assumed the expedition lead and felt responsible for the team's successful ascent.

Hundreds of people climbed Mt. Shasta around the same time each year, following the same route—Avalanche Gulch. Though it had a harrowing moniker, we chose a time of year to summit when the snowpack was still hard enough for crampons and ice axes and for what we hoped would be a fun glissade to the bottom, but the risk of an avalanche was minimal. I had included an old pair of snow pants on the packing list for this very reason. After all, we wanted to have fun after the grueling climb to the top.

I couldn't wait to begin. I figured I wouldn't get a chance to climb much after I got married. My responsibilities as a husband and, hopefully, a father, would be my first priority; and I looked forward to married life. I just hoped Robyn would say yes.

Pete was the most experienced mountaineer in the group. He had been an instructor with the National Outdoor Leadership School and led numerous expeditions in the mountains of Colorado and Wyoming. This would be his first climb from sea level to 14,000 feet in so short a time span—two days. I'd need to watch for signs of impact from the elevation, but I trusted his endurance and stamina after running stride for stride with him in two marathons. He always looked so fresh at each finish; his natural leadership skills and ability to bring out the best in others added another degree of comfort.

Holly Payne, his climbing partner was the only woman on the trip, had limited experience at altitude, and had never camped in snow, but she had been competing in triathlons for five years and rode her bike about a hundred miles each weekend. Endurance was part of her nature. Holly had the will of a lioness, and I believed she'd do well, but I would keep an eye out to make sure.

Matt Gentile was my buddy from MIT. He was the captain of my intramural basketball team over six years earlier when I had the "phantom muscle pull" and the first person to learn about the diagnosis. He had seen me at my worst, and I was anxious to show him the MS hadn't affected me. He had finished several marathons, and I didn't doubt him one bit. His first mountaineering experience was on Mount Washington, the tallest peak on the East Coast at over 6,000 feet, with the fastest recorded wind speed on Earth. He had successfully reached the summit on a weather-challenged day, but this would be his first climb at such a high altitude. He was strong-willed, but his limited experience made me wary and told me I'd need to watch for signs of difficulty.

I had met Bryce May through Gentile. We stayed with him and his wife in Manhattan one weekend while at MIT. He was lean and strong and had just climbed Mount Rainier, so he had experience on snow and at altitude. He had climbed Mount Washington with Matt and was just as determined. I was confident he would make the summit; I would just need to check in with him to make sure all was good.

Matt Riordan's climbing abilities were totally unknown. He was training for a marathon at sea level and had been building his endurance but had never climbed on snow or at altitude. I was most concerned about his performance, but Gentile assured me he was a bull and would make it. I had a great deal of trust in Gentile's judgment. Besides, he told me Riordan was an affable comic and would keep the mood light, a precious commodity on any expedition.

The challenge on Shasta was to climb 3,000 feet in snowshoes with forty-pound packs to 'base camp,' Helen Lake, where we would sleep the first night. We would carry everything we needed for the two days on our backs: food, clothes, ice axes, crampons, snowshoes, tents, and cooking gear. The second day we would climb 4,000 feet to the summit and then descend 7,000 feet back to the cars. The second day would be tougher than a marathon with the weight carried, the altitude climbed, the distance covered, and changing snow conditions. I hadn't told Robyn the specifics of the route before I left because I didn't want to worry her. I just told her we were going to take the same route Brendan and I had successfully climbed the previous year. I wanted to leave her with an optimistic impression of the trip.

Our expedition team met in the town of Shasta at an Italian restaurant and ate a hearty carbo-loaded dinner. The meal provided a chance for Pete and Holly to meet Bryce, Gentile, and Riordan. I was glad everyone was together and getting along—a close team would make it easier to surmount inevitable obstacles on our way to the summit. From a conversation with a local guide, I knew about 45% of the ten thousand people who attempted the summit each year made it, so there was less than a 50/50 chance we'd get to the top.

The next morning, the sunlight roused me from my bag and out of the tent. I was excited. We organized our gear and headed to the parking lot at Bunny Flat. We drove the final five miles, gained 1,000 feet, and arrived at the trailhead. I adjusted my pack to fit snugly on my back, secured my ice axe and snowshoes, and we hit the trail up Avalanche Gulch, named for the frequent masses of snow that careened down its towering slopes. We didn't have to worry. It was late spring and a lot of the winter snow pack had already melted. Plus, our early start allowed us to get on the snow before the intense sun and rising temperatures softened it.

We moved quickly at first, but after a half-hour we began to feel the sun's effects. It happened fast. We started to sink six inches into the softening snow with each step – lumbering like elephants across sand, so we stopped to put on snowshoes. I took the opportunity to add an additional layer of sunscreen. Pete recommended I lather on the sunscreen, even in my nostrils and ears. He said that the intense rays in a snowfield were known to burn those sensitive areas.

With the shoes on, we glided across the snow and organized ourselves into a single file line. The lead person blazed the trail through the softening snow, and then after a hundred strides, fell back to recover. With the team's effort coordinated, we moved rapidly. After an hour, we began to gain altitude. I remember how difficult it was to climb. I took a big step forward and up, but lost half the distance I gained because my shoe slid backward until it bit the snow.

After two hours of sustained climbing, we stopped for a break at 9,000 feet. The altitude and heat had begun to impact our pace and stamina, though we were still an hour ahead of schedule. The group was strong, but I was tired and felt the fatigue as a dull ache deep in my muscles. I threw off my bag and plopped down in the snow to hydrate and eat before the push to Helen Lake.

"Wow, that was a hump. We're what . . . halfway to Helen Lake, which is halfway to the summit," I said, craning my neck to look up at the peak.

"Glad we got that over with," Riordan said to puncture the silence.

We all laughed. I wasn't sure whether I was more beat than the others—I just knew I was worn out. After two more hours, we reached Helen Lake at 10,400 feet. After four hours of continuous movement with forty-pound backpacks on, we finally took them off and scouted a place to pitch our tents—though our first priority was to rehydrate and get water for dinner and the following day's summit and descent. It was the last thing I wanted to do. I was exhausted. I wanted to put up our tent, roll out my sleeping bag, eat a warm snack, and take a well-deserved nap before dinner. Something deep inside me was pleading for me to slow down, but we needed water.

While we had reached Helen Lake, we couldn't just walk to its banks, throw in our filters, and pump our jugs full, because the lake was buried under ten feet of snow. For the next two hours we sat over two stoves, piling snow into small pans. When I finally had enough water in my body and in my jug for the next day's hike, I walked out to a ledge to enjoy the magical sunset over Northern California. I looked out across the valley and fully absorbed the magnitude of our day's accomplishment, but my focus quickly turned to the next day's challenge. I knew the climb to the summit would be difficult, but we'd leave most of our heavy gear at Helen Lake and carry only ten-pound summit packs, shedding nearly thirty pounds of weight. I also knew we wouldn't need snow shoes. Our 2:00 a.m. start meant we would travel when the snow was still hard.

I walked back to camp and made dinner. Freeze-dried red beans and rice. Then I laid out my things for the next day's summit and crawled into my sleeping bag. I dozed off, wanting to get as much sleep as possible. The next morning, my body was stiff, but not more than usual after the previous day's exertion. Dressed in warm layers, I walked out of camp and into the dark morning, guided by the stars and light from my headlamp. I found the trail and got into position to climb the steep grade of the upper gulch to the thumb that stood at nearly 12,500 feet and represented the halfway mark for the climb from Helen Lake to the summit. I checked in with each expedition member while the grade was still relatively flat. The general mood was that it was early and people were sore, but everyone was excited to get going.

I looked uphill and saw the lights of the climbers who had hit the trail two hours earlier. Their tiny stature foreshadowed our early-morning agony. I would need to climb 2,300 feet—like climbing to the top floor of the empire state building twice, just to reach the thumb. The summit was another two miles and 1,700 feet of altitude beyond, not easy with a ten-pound pack on my back, five-pound boots with crampons on each foot, and an ice axe in my uphill hand, which I used like a walking stick to stabilize me on the steep slope and to prevent me from sliding back to Helen Lake if I tripped.

The group moved at the rhythm of ten steps forward, then stopping for a count of ten to rest. The climb was all about pace. I pushed myself hard to stay with the group. The altitude robbed us of slightly less than half of the oxygen we were used to at sea level. I had climbed 1,000 feet of elevation, the last 200 feet beyond my limit, when my body cried for mercy.

"Let's rest here for a minute," I said to Matt, my climbing partner.

"Sure, I could use a break," Gentile said.

I rested on my uphill hand, anchored in place by my ice axe and crampons. I didn't remember this section being so grueling when I had climbed it two years earlier with Brendan. I asked myself why I was struggling so much more than the others. All I could think about was MS.

I looked up and saw that we had at least another thousand feet until we reached the thumb, where the terrain leveled out and I could recover before we tackled Misery Hill. I pushed forward as my body yelled, "STOP!"

The effort to maintain my balance and the altitude lead me to take frequent breaks. The rest of the group continued their pace, while Gentile and I began to fall back. I moved slowly and deliberately. I took five steps and then rested to catch my breath. The pace gave me plenty of time to reflect. MS seemed to be on the move. *What a hell of a time to have an attack*, I thought.

As we crawled up the hill, I began a conversation with MS. I pleaded, *I know I'm out of balance and have pushed way beyond our limits, but please let me summit.*

There was no response, so Gentile and I trudged on. After about two more hours, we arrived below the thumb. I reached the spot where the trail began to level out and saw Pete resting on a rock next to Holly. Bryce and Riordan rested on a ledge above them. I looked toward Pete and said, "How long you been here?"

"About thirty minutes. Good to see you two. How you doing?" Pete asked.

"I'm okay. It feels good to reach the thumb." I wasn't ready to admit I might not be able to make it to the summit.

"Why don't you guys take a break?" Pete suggested, knowing I would not give up easily. I was so close to the top. I took off my pack and sat on a rock. I was relieved to have made it that far but anxious about the distance and elevation that remained. I wasn't sure I could get to the top, but I buried my concern. After ten minutes, Pete stood and put his pack back on. We hiked from the thumb to Red Banks, and I felt good.

My strength returned, and I strayed from the group. I took a less steep track that would allow me to move to Red Bank quicker than the others, but I was alone. I had one goal and it drove me. The panic I'd felt and my pleading conversation with MS faded into the background.

Pete knew better than to let me climb alone, so he broke off to join me. I later found out, before he left the group, he had had a brief conversation with Holly. He asked her to lead the others across the ice field. Holly, who was climbing her first 14er, accepted Pete's challenge and set the pace. He must have known something was up but didn't say anything. He was probably just relieved to see me moving. The trail leveled out above Red Banks, and we took a break for the group to come together for a picture.

After ten minutes, Pete and I packed up and left before the others to start across the flats to Misery Hill. I didn't want to slow them any more than I already had. Pete and I moved well up the switchbacks of Misery Hill. We reached the summit plateau after what seemed like an eternity, our steps slow and heavy. We stood on the flats, and the summit pinnacle came into view.

I rode a wave of euphoria across the snowfield to the base of the summit pinnacle. We scrambled up the final hundred feet, and at eleven o'clock, Pete and I triumphantly stood on top of Mount Shasta. The rest of the team arrived as we finished snapping summit shots. I had a minute to myself while the others caught their breath. I was ecstatic to have reached the summit, but my emotional high was mixed with a sense of impending doom.

I looked down at my watch. It was eleven fifteen. We had roughly eight hours of sunlight to make it from the summit, break down camp, pack our bags, and arrive at the parking lot. It had taken us just under eight hours of strenuous climbing to go from Helen Lake to the summit, and it would take at least six more hours to descend from the summit to the car.

I had done the journey before, so I knew we had enough time, but there wasn't room for error. Before we knew it, we had crossed the summit plateau and were in position to glissade from Red Bank to Helen Lake. We descended the 3,000 feet back to camp at a super-fast clip, because we slid on our butts most of the way, and stood in front of our tent at half past noon. My mountaineering pants were drenched, but since the sun was high in the sky, I appreciated the cool wetness. The ease of the descent from the summit caused me to forget about my difficulty traveling that morning. We broke camp, ate lunch, and at one o'clock, bounded down Avalanche Gulch.

I tried to glissade through the gulch but quickly became bogged down in slush. The elevation wasn't steep enough to carry my speed like it did during the slide from Red Banks to Helen Lake, and the midday sun had softened the snow. It became a slog as we traveled through the Gulch. We trudged downhill and sank six inches in the snow under each step. Travel was grueling because of the soft, slippery conditions and the forty pounds I struggled to balance on my back. My legs were heavy as tree trunks, and I again pleaded with MS to let me make it back to the car.

At about four o'clock, we reached the bottom of the gulch and headed across the flats. My thighs burned from three hours of pounding as I plodded down the mountain. The feeling of exhaustion was more intense than I had ever felt during a marathon. In the years to come, I would feel this same kind of exhaustion after a simple walk from the couch to the kitchen to get a glass of water.

We finally made it to the car, and I set my bag down but struggled to stand. I had a bag of trash that I had accumulated during the trip. I spotted a trashcan, but rather than walk over and toss it out, I stood like a statue. I couldn't drag myself to the can. I had no strength in my legs; I was wiped out and completely delirious. I asked Riordan how he was doing. He responded with something like, "Dude, I fucking don't want to do that again anytime soon."

Bryce, Gentile, and I laughed in spite of hardly having the energy for even that. Fifteen minutes later Pete and Holly arrived and put their bags down. They wore looks of dazed exhaustion. We didn't celebrate. We didn't really say much of anything. After a prolonged break, I threw out my trash and packed the car. I hugged Pete, said good-bye to Holly, and wished them a safe ride back to San Francisco. Riordan, Gentile, Bryce and I slowly got in the car for the two-hour drive to the airport in Redding.

Very little was said during the drive. I'm sure the others appreciated being able to sit and relax. I was pleased to have accomplished my mission but was having a hard time admitting that something the opposite of magic had happened on that mountain. My body wasn't right. I remembered pleading with the MS to allow me to reach the summit. When I heard no response, I put my head down and bulled my way through the climb, but there was no denying my performance had slipped. I was only thirty-three and my body should have been able to reach new endurance thresholds when pushed to the limit. That clearly wasn't the case. It seemed as if my physical vitality had peaked. The thought sent a chill of fear radiating through me. Shasta would be the last 14er I would ever climb.

PART IV
THE FALL

15

MY ENGAGEMENT... TO MS

It was one thing to live in denial of MS as a single man, but if I got married, the woman of my dreams would have to marry the MS, too. Taking the vow "for better or for worse, during good times and bad, in sickness and in health, 'till death do us part" took on a very different meaning for me at the age of thirty-three. I was uncertain that I could share a long, "healthy" life with anyone. Was it fair to ask Robyn?

How would I hold up? Would I stay in the A plus group, or would I be in a wheelchair by forty? I had no way to predict the future. I only knew that I was in love.

I wanted to do something big for Robyn. I booked a weekend at Bacara Resort and Spa, a five-star resort on the Pacific Coast just outside Santa Barbara. When we woke up in the largest, most comfortable bed we had ever slept in, I reminded Robyn at least half a dozen times that I wanted to walk the beach before lunch. Later, Robyn told me I was acting like a total freak—jumpy, spacey, and distracted, but she went along with it.

We headed for a secluded bluff that overlooked the ocean—it was the perfect place for a once-in-a-lifetime event. I dropped to one knee with my right hand in my coat pocket, kneeled under the oak tree, and broke the ice: "I'm so happy that I finally asked you out after sitting in your chair for a year. I took a chance you'd say yes, and we've been together since. I'm thankful."

"Me too," she said.

"You bring out the best in me, and I want to spend the rest of my life with you."

Robyn's blue eyes opened wide and her face softened, but when I finished, she started to laugh uncontrollably—not the response I expected, and I tried to maintain my composure. I couldn't tell if she was laughing at me or the situation. I didn't want to be derailed, so I picked up the pace. I pulled the ring from my pocket and offered it to her.

"Robyn, will you marry me?"

I remained on one knee for what seemed an eternity. My eyes fixed on hers. I watched and waited. She couldn't stop laughing, and I began to feel self-conscious down on one knee. I stood and forced the point. "So what do you think? Will you marry me?"

"YES, of course I'll marry you."

We both laughed, I moved toward her, and we embraced. My body tingled from head to toe—a mix of adrenalin and endorphins. I'm not sure if the feeling was from joy or because the circulation finally returned to my legs, but it felt good; and in the years ahead, during the most severe MS attacks, I would come to miss that feeling.

Two weeks after our engagement, we traveled to Newfoundland to visit Robyn's family. We crisscrossed the island, west to east, from Deer Lake to St. John's and visited her parents first, who had recently returned home after living in New Hampshire and Maine for the previous thirty years. We also spent time with her grandmother and her aunts, uncles, and cousins, whom Robyn hadn't seen in nearly ten years.

I appreciated the long hours of conversation around campfires and kitchen tables, and felt the tremendous sense of family and community for which Newfoundlers were known. I liked how her family lived. They didn't have superfluous material possessions vying for their attention, and rather than spend time watching television or sitting in front of a computer, they spent their time talking with each other— telling stories and laughing. This was the kind of family life I hoped to create with Robyn.

◆

A week into the trip, I felt congested. We took a hike in the woods. I hoped the exercise would help clear my head, but it didn't. My symptoms worsened: skull-splitting headache, tingling in my hands and feet, as well as stiffness in my legs that affected how I walked. My gait became jerky and disjointed. I had no idea what was happening. I put on my running shoes and took a five-mile jog.

The run didn't loosen me up as I'd hoped. Instead, my body continued to seize. I became increasingly frustrated as I ran. Rather than free me, I felt imprisoned with each stride. It was the last time I would ever run that distance.

My condition deteriorated. I had exhaustion deep in my bones that I couldn't sleep off and had trouble breathing as well as a tingling in my fingers and toes. Robyn called her dad, who came to the cabin. They rushed me to an urgent care hospital. I was admitted and the doctor showed me to a private room and gave me a sleep aid. I spent the night under a doctor's supervision. I woke the next morning and still had a headache but felt a little better after a solid night's sleep. Robyn came to get me, and I was released.

Later that week, I sat around a campfire with Robyn, her parents, her Aunt Carmalita, Uncle Geo, and cousin Christopher. We tried to make light of my emergency room experience. It was the best way we knew how to deal with the circumstance. My congestion and muscle stiffness persisted but weren't as bad as the night after my run. I threw another log in the fire, when something hit me.

"Bernie, what kind of wood is that?" I asked Robyn's father.

"It's alder—that's the tree that covers the island."

The news was inconsequential to most, but I happened to be allergic to alder trees. Since the trees blanketed the island, the air was filled with its pollen. I had discovered I was allergic thirty years earlier, as a boy in Vermont. This was the first time I saw the link between my environment and the onset of MS symptoms.

When we got back to LA, Robyn called Andy and told him what had happened in Newfoundland. She told him my symptoms: the tingling, stiffness, and splitting headache. He prescribed a round of steroids.

That fall, I worked hard to stay in top shape. My equilibrium and balance were continuing to deteriorate due to the MS. As the result of hidden damage to my nervous system, I wasn't able to run outdoors so I joined a gym around the block from work and found I couldn't even run on the treadmill while gripping the handrails. I rode the stationary bike instead. I hoped the exercise would allow me to maintain my strength and endurance, and improve my balance, which had become less and less stable.

I remember one night's workout. I tried my hardest not to wobble as I walked through the gym. Fear began to grip me: fear of tripping, fear of others noticing me waver, fear of losing my position at work. I hoped the impact to my balance and equilibrium weren't permanent and that my body would fully recover like it had before.

I was concerned but stayed tight-lipped about the progression of the MS because I felt nothing good would come of telling others, only shame and regret. Like I wasn't doing enough to fight it, or that it was somehow winning. I fought to stay one step ahead of the team at work, hoping that my colleagues would not notice my struggles.

I continued to work out three times each week, believing exercise would improve my condition. I rode the stationary bike twice a week at the gym, and on Saturday rode my mountain bike, traveling up the Pacific Coast to my refuge at Sycamore State Park. But it was there, on my bike, that I felt the symptoms of MS most acutely. I didn't want to fall and learned to carefully mount and dismount, both in the gym and outdoors. I rode with increasing caution as my leg strength waned and my balance continued to waver.

♦

In late fall, I rode with Brendan and another buddy, Lars, again at Sycamore Canyon. Lars had become part of our Saturday morning ritual a few weeks earlier. He was a strong rider and a madman on descents. I never asked Brendan why he invited him. I didn't want to hear that Brendan needed someone to challenge him because I no longer could.

We started the ride together, but as we rode out the canyon floor, we separated. Lars and Brendan took a path up a 2,000-foot technically-challenging single track. I had lost the strength, stamina, and balance to successfully navigate the trail, and rather than ride with them and risk a fall, I continued out the flat canyon floor and ascended a more moderate route. I decided to ride the less dangerous route after a conversation with Robyn, who had become increasingly concerned about my welfare.

I crossed paths with Brendan and Lars at the halfway point, as they descended the Guadalsco trail and I began to climb it. The route was challenging, but the path was wide and in good enough condition for me to successfully navigate. I was still able to ride the trail and savored the short-lived feeling of accomplishment at the top. Though separated for the majority of the ride, passing Brendan and Lars left me with the sense that we were experiencing the ride together. This was critical for my delicate psyche, and it allowed us to talk about the shared experience on the forty-five minute drive home. I was thankful they were okay with me riding with them.

We did the same ride a few weeks later. We separated at our usual place, and I pushed myself hard to maintain my pace so we would meet at the Guadalasco Trailhead. About a mile after we split, I had to stop to rest because I was overheated and felt like I was spinning out of control. I had ridden this trail many times before and never had to get off my bike to rest. I stopped to dismount and felt humiliated. I struggled to stand. I had felt that sensation before, in college, going to bed after too much to drink—the bed spins.

I sat on the soft dirt of the Sycamore Canyon Trail. When I tried to look up at a big green oak tree, I had to stop and quickly look down at the dirt and close my eyes. Sitting on the ground with my eyes shut helped to stop the spins. I was worried; I had taken the Rebif for the previous five months. Robyn injected me with the drug three times each week, but I didn't feel any better; I felt worse. This was hard to take as the injections cost my insurance more than a thousand dollars every month. I hopped back on my bike and met my riding buddies.

"How long you been waiting?" I asked when I arrived.

"We just got here a minute ago. Everything all right? Thought you might have had a spill," Brendan said, studying my face.

"I didn't fall, but I needed to get off my bike to fix my chain."

I didn't want to tell them the truth and threaten my Saturday ride. I couldn't admit to myself what Brendan and Lars were well aware of—my performance was slipping.

16

BREAKING POINT: PLAYING THE MS CARD

In the winter of 2004, I struggled physically but was able to perform at work and remained hopeful that MS wouldn't affect me professionally. I was managing software developers on an application design in Santa Monica and had to travel to Sapient's New Delhi office to make sure the team could finish the job.

During my first trip to New Delhi, I was happy to make it through my two weeks unscathed by the kind of stories associated with travel in India. I didn't get sick. I didn't get hassled. Our team was on track, and I was continuing to advance within the company.

It wasn't just Sapient I aimed to please—Robyn was waiting for me in California so we could fly east the next day to attend our engagement party that her sister Ray had planned in Rye, New Hampshire. I did everything I could to make sure I was on that flight. She wasn't too happy to hear I had planned to cut it so close. Most of her family and close childhood friends planned to attend. I'd be there— just after I flew around the world first. No problem, right?

Wrong. I arrived at the airport three and a half hours early, an hour earlier than normal, even for a post 9-11 international flight. I strode to the counter to get my boarding pass, but when I reached into my coat pocket for my passport, I found only my hotel receipt and a paper clip. No passport.

Alarmed, I stood off to the side of the line and riffled through my clothes and carry-on, then paged through my travel papers. I knew the passport accompanied the two photos of Robyn that I always carried with me. I had seen the photos and the passport the previous day when I packed, but that morning I only found the photos. I ran through scenarios of where I might have put my passport and concluded it must have been stolen.

I wasn't allowed on the plane without it and was told I would need to go to the embassy for a travel letter. I wasn't sure what that meant, but I knew it probably wasn't as easy as showing up at the embassy window and asking. I went to the embassy and found out that what I really needed was a replacement.

I spent the entire day, thousands of ruppees, and took half a dozen cab rides trying to get a passport photo, fill out a police report, and withdraw the money I needed for the embassy to create a new one. More than ten hours later and thousands of rupees lighter, I did something I thought I would never do. I turned to the lady at the Embassy and told a complete stranger the secret I'd tried for years to hide: "I have multiple sclerosis and take shots daily. I'm out of medicine, so I need a new passport and an exit visa to return home immediately."

The embassy agent turned to her coworker, told him about my predicament, and they worked to make my replacement. I checked back into my hotel for a few hours rest before my early morning flight. I ordered some dinner, and then I called Robyn to let her know I had changed my plans, that I would fly west through London rather than east through Hong Kong and arrive in Boston Saturday afternoon before the party. It was the best I could do. She was more than baffled to hear I was still in Delhi and not on a plane.

"Are you alright?" she asked, her voice full of panic.

"Yeah, it's a long story. I'll tell you all about it when I see you."

"Make sure you set an alarm. And be safe. I love you."

"I love you, too."

I slept most of the fourteen-hour trip to Boston, except for the two and a half hours I waited in London Heathrow airport to clear US customs, but I made it to Boston and then Rye in time for the party. My body was confused after twenty hours of travel through thirteen time zones. When I met Robyn's childhood friends, I'm not sure of the impression I made beyond a warm greeting and a brief recounting of my trip. I was in no state to interact with people. After an hour and a half of hellos, hugs, and handshakes, I found myself on the living room couch, sitting alone in the dark, and fell asleep.

The next day, Robyn told me that during the party she was in the kitchen when a friend asked her where I was. She did a quick scan of the room but couldn't find me. Concerned, she asked her brother-in-law if he knew where I was. He told her to check the living room. Robyn knew that room wasn't in use for the party, so she went to investigate and found me sitting upright on the couch, fast asleep. She roused me and brought me upstairs to bed. Robyn and I didn't talk about my lost passport. Like me, she conveniently denied that my condition would alter our lives. We were getting married, after all, and we had not invited MS to the wedding.

During a trip to the dry cleaner two weeks later in LA, Robyn was given the passport that I thought had been stolen. The dry cleaner found it in the back pocket of a pair of pants and returned it with my pressed clothes.

This was the first time my mental faculties were being affected by MS. I should have recalled the last time I had seen my passport and thought to look in my pants pocket as I frantically riffled through my things at the airport, but I couldn't because the MS was starting to cloud my thinking. Even then, confronted with proof, I still remained in denial.

I knew I had Robyn by my side, but I still didn't know how to ask her for help.

♦

In the spring before we were married, I created colossal to-do lists so that at the end of the day I could feel a sense of accomplishment. The lists allowed me to look past the MS symptoms I was experiencing—the brain fog, reduced strength, tingling in my hands and feet, and feelings of imbalance when I walked.

I tried hard to remain one step ahead of MS when I worked, when I struggled to exercise, and even for the fifteen minutes when Robyn injected me with the drug three nights a week, but my veneer of invincibility started to show cracks. I wondered how long it would be until the foundation I had worked so hard to build started to crumble. I dealt with my circumstances the way I always had—I dug in, lowered my head, and worked harder. The more I had to do, the less I had to feel—a convenient way to cope.

Robyn filled her life with the same level of activity. She returned to school to complete her degree, after a ten-year hiatus, because she was ready for a career change and needed a new challenge. She reduced her hours at the salon to accommodate her studies. Between school and work, she averaged at least fifty-hour weeks.

In the little free time she had, Robyn made arrangements for our wedding. We chose to get married in Rye, New Hampshire, because it was outside of Portsmouth, where she used to live and where her sister still lived. The location was also close for our friends and family who were scattered from Philadelphia to Newfoundland. Planning a wedding from three thousand miles away added to the difficulty of the task, but we wanted to make it easy for our close family and friends to attend.

Robyn shouldered the responsibilities, making all the arrangements on her own, without the assistance of a wedding planner—relying on her sister to help decide on a venue. I was grateful she took on the challenges of wedding planning, because I couldn't. I left the office most nights with barely enough stamina to work out twice a week, though I still clung to my invincible persona on Saturday rides with Brendan and Lars.

When I got home after work, I sat on the couch and fell asleep. I continued to walk through life with blinders on. I was engaged to be married, had my dream in hand, and didn't want to face the reality of my condition.

My body soon forced me to look inward. That winter, I finally faced the truth. My strength and balance were getting worse. I felt it most acutely on long weekend rides, as it became more of a struggle to stay on the bike. I remember one Saturday morning at the end of a ride at Sycamore Canyon, when I rode the final two-mile spin along the flat trail to the car and struggled to keep my balance. My legs clutched the middle bar to keep contact with the centerline, so I didn't lose control and veer off the trail, and my arms were exhausted as they fought to hold onto the bike.

When I got home, I was barely able to maneuver my bike into the apartment. As I brought it to the third floor, I bumped into railings and furniture, like I was drunk. When I arrived at Robyn's door, I greeted her with a big hug, relieved to be home. I imagined she was relieved to see me, too. My rides were becoming longer and longer, and what once had taken me two hours, now took me twice as long. Though she never said anything about my rides, she probably wondered when she would have to rescue me from a crash.

I put my stuff down and dove into bed for a two-hour nap. When I woke, my body was still completely fatigued. I had biked twenty miles and gained fifteen hundred feet. The numbers provided some reassurance, but they also scared me. I could ride ten more miles and gain twice as much altitude in a third less time just eight months earlier.

That night Robyn and I talked about the ride. She initiated the conversation, as usual. If she didn't ask, I would not have shared anything about what happened.

"How was the ride today?"

"Good. We rode twenty miles and gained fifteen hundred feet."

"How did Brendan do?"

"He's a mutant."

"That's not really what I asked. Did he ride well?"

"Neither of us fell today, if that's what you're asking."

"It's not; I remember you telling me how you two used to race up the hill. Today you came home so tired; I figured you might have raced."

I wanted to avoid the issue of my performance, but one of the things I cherished most about our relationship was our honesty. It was time for me to fess up.

"Actually, we didn't really ride together today. I met him at the halfway point because he took a more technically difficult trail than me."

"Really . . . why didn't you ride together?"

"I rode the Canyon floor and stayed on wider fire road trails."

She stared at me, concerned. "Why?"

I was irritated by the question, but I knew Robyn wouldn't allow me to avoid answering. I had been with Robyn long enough to realize her questions came from her heart. She spoke with love and support; I knew her concern was for my well-being.

"My balance and strength aren't as good as they used to be, and it's hard to stay on the single-track trails that Brendan rides, so we ride separate, but we check in at the halfway point to make sure we're both okay."

She stared at me. "What are we going to do? I thought the Rebif was supposed to stop the decline, if not help you get stronger?"

"I hoped the same thing, but it's not. Things are getting worse."

"I agree, you've been wobbling around the apartment, and ever since you started taking that stuff you fall asleep on the couch at 8:30. It scares me."

"Me too."

"What do you think we should do about it?"

"There are four different medications. Andy said that Rebif is the strongest, if I can handle it. It doesn't look like I can handle it."

"No, it doesn't."

Later that month, we met with Andy and explained my deteriorating balance and leg strength. He was understanding and wanted the best for me. He listened to what I had to say and suggested I try Avonex, a new medication. He handed me a prescription and told me he would work out the details with my insurance company. He said I would need to wait several weeks before I started with the Avonex, to let my body process the Rebif first. Robyn and I both hoped the medication explained my deteriorating symptoms since our trip to Newfoundland.

A month later, the Avonex arrived. There were five neatly packed syringes with two-inch needles protruding from each. The drug needed to be injected deep into the muscle, which explained the needle length. With every new medication came a new nurse to walk me through the first injection. The night of my first Avonex injection, I left work early to meet the nurse at 5:30 at our apartment. I scheduled the meeting before Robyn returned home from work, because I wanted to take greater responsibility for my injections and reduce the burden on her.

At 6:30 Robyn returned from work. "You're home early," she said.

"I came home about an hour ago and met the nurse to do the Avonex shot. She just left," I said confidently.

"What!? You did the injection without me? I wanted to be here to make sure I'm up to speed on the new medication. You need to include me in stuff like that."

I thought I was doing a good thing. I wanted to reduce the burden she felt to care for me, but my confidence vaporized when I realized I should have included her. I sat on the couch in silence and fell asleep. At 8:00, I groggily headed to bed. I woke a few hours later from a deep sleep calling Robyn's name from the bedroom. She jumped off the couch and hurried to my side.

"I'm freezing and I have to use the bathroom," I slurred.

Robyn stood beside me trying to figure out what I was saying and more importantly what was happening. She felt my forehead—my face was covered in sweat. She quickly ran her hands across my t-shirt, pillow, and sheets; they were all soaked. She knew something was terribly wrong. She watched as I struggled to swing my legs to the floor to stand. They wouldn't work, so I had to use my arms. With my feet on the ground, I struggled to stand. I stood for a moment but began to waver. I thought I just needed to gather myself and wake up before I made my way to the bathroom, but I couldn't steady myself. Off-balance, I fell back into bed.

"Oh God, are you okay!?"

I strained to respond. When I opened my mouth, I couldn't speak, my mouth didn't work. I only slurred.

"I'm here, are you all right, what can I do?" she pleaded.

I was only able to mumble that I needed to go to the bathroom, so Robyn made sure my legs were securely positioned on the floor and said, "On the count of three, I'll lift you up. Ready? One, two, three."

Robyn lifted me out of bed, and I held on to her and we slowly made our way to the bathroom. Robyn held me like a Marine carrying an injured comrade. After what seemed an eternity, I arrived at the toilet. Robyn lowered me to the seat. There was no way I was going to be able to stand.

"Do you need me to stand here while you go?"

"No, I'm okay."

Robyn nervously left the bathroom and waited outside the door. I desperately wanted to regain my self-respect. I couldn't understand what was going on. I thought about what might have triggered the attack. I went through my routine before going to sleep, when it hit me. I injected the Avonex for the first time. With the thought of the injection lingering, I told Robyn I was ready to go back to bed.

Robyn helped me to my feet. "I'm freezing," I told her.

"You're shaking. Let's change your clothes."

We headed back to bed. When I was safely in bed, Robyn went to the closet and got me a change of clothes. She had taken a towel from the bathroom. She helped me stand, wiped off the sweat, and changed my clothes. When I was dry and in a new set of clothes, she helped me into bed and then wrapped me in blankets and held me tight to make sure I was warm.

She told me later that this went on all night—cold . . . hot . . . cold . . . hot. She said in between each cold and hot spell, I would pass out. Robyn said she just lay there next to me making sure I was breathing and wondering if she should call an ambulance. Before dawn, Robyn said she finally passed out.

The next morning, I rose from bed and was able to walk to the bathroom on my own. It was a major victory, though I still wobbled. I kissed Robyn on the forehead before I left the room.

She opened her eyes. "You're up," she said, surprised. "How do you feel?"

"I feel alright, a bit tired, but I need to get into the office. How'd you sleep?"

"I didn't. I was up most of the night to make sure you were breathing. This shit almost had me calling the EMTs."

We stared at each other for one awkward moment.

"You need to call Andy today and let him know what happened. Enough is fucking enough." Robyn didn't swear unless she was terrified or enraged. She was both.

I promised her I would call Andy. Aside from the morning of the diagnosis and the day of my mother's imagined Mafia threat, it had been the scariest moment of my life. I had never felt more helpless. It was like I was paralyzed but fully conscious. I never wanted to feel that way again, and I was willing to give just about any different drug a try to make sure I wouldn't.

17

CRASHING THE THRESHOLD

A month before we were married, I started another medication. My hands tingled, my feet were losing feeling, and I was losing my balance more and more when I walked. I hoped that the dance classes Robyn and I had just completed would pay off in muscle memory at the reception. I wanted to avoid the embarrassment and the whispers about my unsteady steps.

"That's right, he has MS."

Over the previous nine months, I had begun to share the diagnosis with a wider circle of friends and family. It was no longer possible to keep my secret. It was obvious my health suffered. Robyn and I hoped the change in medication, as well as relaxing on the beach for two weeks during our honeymoon, would provide the shift I needed to improve my condition.

The night before the wedding, in bed in a hotel in New Hampshire, I thought about ways to sneak over and see Robyn at her sister's house for a secret rendezvous, but didn't want to jinx us. I had enough on my mind, considering the magnitude of the next day. I wasn't worried about the lifelong commitment I was about to make, or even if I would remember my vows and could dance—though those thoughts had consumed me lately. I worried again about providing for Robyn if the MS got worse.

How long would it be until I needed a walker or a wheelchair? I had been able to keep the MS at bay for the first six years after the diagnosis, but everything had changed since our engagement, especially my vision of the future with Robyn: a life of prosperity and abundance; a family, kids and a dog. We would live in a nice house on a half-acre in a safe neighborhood. We would send our kids to the best schools and take a few vacations each year to seaside or mountaintop resorts. The vision didn't include MS and I wondered how long my body would keep the promises I was about to make.

The next morning, I woke and met my parents for breakfast in the hotel dining room. As I ate, I looked through the picture window at the salt marsh that led into Portsmouth Harbor under a sunny, clear sky. The day had the makings of the best day of my life. I pulsed with excitement. I couldn't wait to begin my life with Robyn, even with all those questions weighing heavily on my mind.

Before lunch, my brother Pete held a private yoga session for a half dozen of our guests. We gathered around him on the lawn, in front of the hotel, next to an apple tree in full bloom. The pink and white flowers were a sea of color. The temperature was in the high seventies, and a warm offshore breeze blew. It felt perfect, except for one thing.

I had tingling and loss of sensation and strength in my extremities again, and couldn't even do tree pose. My balance didn't allow me to stand on one leg. Rather than continue to thrash and draw attention, I moved toward the tree and grabbed a branch. I stood in the back of the group and hoped the others hadn't seen me struggle.

After yoga, I ate lunch with my family then went back to my room and practiced my vows. I wanted to get all the way through them once from memory, and then take a nap, but each time I attempted, I had to look down at the paper before I reached the end. I had wanted to impress Robyn, but my mind wasn't cooperating. I was stressed and grasping for the words, so I stopped to rest. I figured the pastor would prompt me if I got stuck. The thought consoled me, and I dozed off to sleep.

When I woke, I showered and dressed, struggling only when I put on cufflinks. I fumbled for a few minutes, finding it difficult to line up the holes in the shirt cuffs and slide the prong through. Somehow, I managed to get them on and saved myself the humiliation when Brendan knocked to take me to the church. I quickly scanned the room and grabbed my vows to review on the drive, tucking them in my pocket.

We arrived at the church and walked to the patio where my parents were waiting with Pete. As I passed the empty pews, it struck me that in less than an hour, I would leave with Robyn, my wife.

"How are you?" Pete asked.

"Good. Nervous, but I think I'm ready."

"I have the ring in my pocket," Pete reassured me.

When the Reverend gathered Pete and me, my parents took the cue to leave. As my mom passed, I remembered the letter she had written three years earlier, the day I asked Robyn for a date. It was one of my mom's greatest dreams for me to find a partner, and in thirty minutes, I would be married to the woman who had unlocked my heart, thanks in part to my mom's encouragement and guidance.

The reverend confirmed Pete had the ring and reminded us to breathe and not lock our knees. Then he looked at me. "Jon, you have your vows committed to memory, right?"

My heart sank. I looked at him, stricken.

"Aahh . . . yeah . . . pretty much."

He smiled. "I'm just kidding. I will feed you your lines—just repeat after me."

I entered the chapel and noticed it was full of familiar faces. In the background, a violin played. I took my place at the altar and stood at attention. My eyes focused on the back wall and expectantly awaited the arrival of my bride. The violin went silent, and the organ roared to life. Robyn entered the church and I thought *this is my beautiful life, and the beautiful woman walking down the aisle is going to be my wife.*

My heart pounded and I shifted my weight to my toes, watching her turn the corner and walk down the aisle with her father. When they reached the altar, he kissed her, offered me his daughter's hand, shook my hand, and then gave me a confident nod, as if to say, "Here you go, bud, all the best."

The ceremony went off without a hitch, and my MS remained a silent witness. The reverend kept his promise and gave me my vows word-for-word. When I finished, Robyn wiped the sweat from my forehead and repeated her vows. When she said "in sickness and in health," I heard a hitch in her voice but knew our union was official.

The significance of those five simple words hit me. I would never again shoulder the pain, loss, and grief alone; and the vow I had taken behind the woodpile thirty years earlier vanished. I no longer needed to be strong and rely only on myself to stay safe. I had Robyn. We exchanged rings, kissed, and walked out of the church. Robyn and I savored the moment. "We did it!" Robyn said, as she put her arms around me.

"Yes, we did," I said and drew her in for another kiss.

After the drive to the hotel, and an hour and a half of photos, we waited at the door of the Grand Ballroom to be announced. My legs were tired from being on my feet, and they started to lose responsiveness. My movements were jerky and strained.

As we stood ready to enter the reception, I worried a hundred people would be focused on my every move. I didn't know how evident my MS appeared. It didn't matter how well I knew the dance moves if my body couldn't cooperate. I told myself I just needed to make it through the song, so I could sit and rest while we ate. I tried to make another deal with the MS, but my request fell on deaf ears. Before the doors swung open, I whispered in Robyn's ear, "I don't feel up to the dance."

"Alright," she said, without a hint of protest.

The doors swung open, and Robyn and I walked to the center of the dance floor. As we stood in position and waited for our song to begin, I whispered in her ear again. "Thank you."

We abandoned our carefully choreographed dance in favor of the waltz-like move I picked up during my two years of cotillion in middle school. Our bodies moved around the dance floor. I became lost in the music as I held Robyn. At one point, I looked toward my mom and gave her a look of gratitude. As the music ended, our guests clapped and we took our seats. I breathed deeply, knowing the hard parts—the vows and dance—were over. It was time to relax and enjoy the night.

After the toasts, my MS left the room, and I found a wave of adrenalin that I rode as we danced with our guests, cut the cake, and walked to each table to thank our guests.

At eleven thirty, the night officially ended, but rather than retire for the evening, two dozen of our friends took over the hotel bar and piano lounge. I'm not sure who paid the piano player to stick around, but for the next two hours, we sang songs from our school days. I couldn't have imagined the night with a better ending.

After last call, one of my buddies bought a couple bottles of wine, and a dozen partiers followed us to our room to continue the good times. I should have ended the night there, but I got swept up. As we stood at the door of our bridal suite in the tower room of the hotel, the group cheered me on to carry Robyn over the threshold. Robyn initially resisted but finally relented. That was when I knew we had gone too far.

Caught up in the moment, I unlocked the door with my card key, and then bent down and cradled Robyn in my arms. She held on to me with her arms around my neck. I realized then that I had made a commitment my body couldn't keep, and my arms and legs gave way. I panicked and tried to catch myself, but it was too late. They didn't have the strength or stamina to hold her, much less walk three feet, and Robyn fell.

Surrounded by my buddies, I saw my bride on the ground. I looked into her eyes and saw pain. It wasn't a physical ache from her fall to the floor; it was an emotional hurt mixed with embarrassment. I hadn't seen that look before, and I never wanted to see it again. The group went silent, but rather than add to the grief, Robyn jumped up and tried to console the group.

"I'm fine, no big deal. Everyone come in! Who has the wine?" she said, laughing.

It was in that moment I knew how right we were. I would rely on her understanding in the face of challenge again and again in the years to come.

18

A "FRIENDLY" FAMILY INTERVENTION

Three months after we were married, my family came to visit. My parents flew in from Philadelphia, and Pete flew in from San Francisco. We bought a new house two months prior and were having work done, so they couldn't stay at our place. We met Pete and my parents at a hotel nearby. I remember walking into my parent's room with Robyn and seeing my mom seated on the bed and Pete and my dad seated around a small table. There was an air of formality, and I knew something was up.

After a brief yet warm welcome and a few pleasantries, my father asked how things were going. I assumed he was referring to the new house.

"We're excited about the new place," I said. "It feels good to be all moved in and to have a place of our own. It needs work, but it's perfect; can't wait for you to see it."

"We are looking forward to it, but I'm more interested to hear how you're feeling," my dad continued.

I paused, feeling the tension in the room. Small talk was not going to cut it.

"I feel okay. I've been taking the Copaxone and going to the gym a few times a week."

Up to this point, my mother had been quiet, which was typical as she tried to get a feel for the situation, but I was suspicious of Pete's silence. He always contributed to the conversation, but his reluctance to talk made me anxious. With my father in the lead, I began to feel like this was less of a friendly family visit and more of an intervention.

I looked over at Robyn. "Robyn gives me a shot every night."

"We're glad to hear you are taking the medication, but we're concerned. At the wedding, your balance was off, and your movements were slow and delayed. We haven't seen you like this. Is this how things are for you now?"

"I'm struggling," I said as I looked at Robyn.

My father continued. "Thanksgiving was the last time we saw you before the wedding, and ever since, your condition has declined significantly. We're worried and don't like to see you like this. We want to know if there's anything we can do to help?"

"Dad, we're concerned, too. We've tried all of the conventional treatments, all of the medications, and two of them kicked my ass. Remember the story of Robyn walking me to the bathroom?"

"That was scary," my mom finally interjected.

"We eat pretty well, and I exercise a few times a week."

"We know you take good care of yourself, Jon, that's not the issue. We just don't like to see your condition decline, and we want to talk about what can be done to turn things around."

I shifted in my seat, deflated by the inquisition.

"Dad, I'm not sure there is anything we can do. Multiple sclerosis is a degenerative disease that leads to gradual decline, even paralysis. My condition has declined significantly since we saw you last, and maybe my relapsing-remitting MS has evolved into secondary-progressive MS."

"How can you check that?" my dad asked.

"I'm not sure, but we will check with Dr. Woo next time we see him. I think I have an appointment in early January, right, babe?"

I turned to Robyn, grateful, as she jumped in to speak.

"Yeah, January; I know easier said than done, but try not to worry," she said. "I mean, we are worried too, but we're trying our best to figure out what to do to stop this. We have not only seen the neurologist but also Jon's general practitioner, Ernie Prudente. Unfortunately, they all say the same stupid thing. Nothing! They say, *This is not unexpected, and to continue to do your best.*"

Robyn paused and took a deep breath while my family sat and listened, stunned.

Robyn continued to vent her frustration. "They all say Jon looks good, but they don't have to live with it every day."

"Wow, I didn't know you were struggling so much," my dad said.

Pete finally broke his silence. "Jon, you know I love you. You're my only brother, and it hurts me to see you like this. I am going down to this raw vegan retreat center after the first of the year. The place has an amazing track record for turning around health conditions like cancer."

"What are their results with MS?"

"I'm not sure but will look into it while I'm there. I will do anything for you to get better," Pete said, as his voice cracked and his eyes welled.

"I don't want to end up in a wheelchair," I said, willing to give anything a try.

19
NAIL IN THE COFFIN

As we finished the remodel during the fall of 2004, the MS attacks continued. I had lived with the disease for close to eight years, and it was now on full display. MS was awake and thriving. I was reminded each time I went to the bathroom. Now, I had to sit. My legs were too weak, and I didn't have the strength or stamina to keep my balance. I had always been told by popular culture that real men stood to piss and now I felt like less of a man. I was also feeling the effects of the disease on my manhood when Robyn and I made love. I suffered from erectile dysfunction; it was a hard pill to swallow.

One Sunday afternoon, on my way to the living room to watch a basketball game, I tumbled down the remodeled stairs. It happened so fast. Due to the increasing numbness in my legs, I overshot the fourth stair. I landed hard on my right elbow and hip, and then slid down the remaining three steps to the bottom. Robyn ran from the kitchen when she heard the crack of bone on bamboo.

"Holy crap! Are you okay?" she asked.

"Give me a minute."

I tentatively stood and placed weight on my legs, carefully scanning my body. My elbow throbbed. I flexed to make sure it worked; it did. I stood there for a minute and shifted my full weight onto my right leg; pain shot through my hip. I leaned on Robyn and gingerly hobbled around the kitchen, carefully placing more weight on my hip with each step. It held.

"I think I'm okay," I said. "My elbow and hip bore the brunt of the fall. Neither feel broken, but they're real sore."

Robyn walked me to the chair by the TV and brought me an ice pack.

"Stay in the chair, please."

I followed her advice. I watched the teams battle it out on the court, and my attention was diverted from the pain. TV was my opiate, and my time in front of it grew. During the holiday season, work was slow. The automotive client I worked for was shut down between Christmas and New Year's, so I didn't have project demands. I had more free time than usual, but free time, I would learn, could be dangerous.

To keep busy, I decided to complete a training requirement for my job and enrolled in an online project management course. I had served as a project manager at Sapient for the previous seven and a half years, probably longer than 95% of project managers in the company, so I assumed I would ace it. Halfway through a review of the materials, I knew I was in trouble. My mind went in circles as it tried to keep ideas straight. I was perplexed. What were once clear concepts about project management at Sapient had become confusing.

After I reviewed the material, I took the online exam to receive course credit. I was shocked with the result: sixty-three. I needed seventy to pass. I sat at my desk with my head in my hands and stared at the screen. I wasn't sure what to do.

I was glad the exam was online because it was graded on the spot by the computer, and no one except my career manager, who was emailed my score, would see my failure. How would he react? How might this impact my employment? I reviewed each question and was given the correct answer. Thankfully, I had as many chances as I needed to pass the test. If I could pass it that same day, the system would only submit my most recent score. There was a chance my manager would not see my failing grade.

After I reviewed the material, I retook the exam. I was pleased that the questions were exactly the same, but I felt as unsure of the answers as the first time and anxiously hit the submit button. I stared out the window while I waited for my score.

I worried what my manager would do if I failed again, and worse, I wondered if I was losing my mind. Since the diagnosis, I was led to believe that the MS wouldn't affect my cognitive abilities. My mind had always been a source of strength; my ability to think rationally and recall what I had read had allowed me to excel at work and in school. Once, when I was studying abroad in France, I took a quiz on French government and was questioned if I cheated because I had identified all the areas of government and didn't misspell a word. I assured my teacher that I didn't cheat and had spent a lot of time studying. After taking the test at Sapient, I was no longer sure I had this recall ability.

I looked back at the screen to see my test score, and it validated my worst fear. I had scored sixty-nine and had failed the course again. How could this be? I had practiced project management daily for the previous seven and a half years. I should have known the concepts, but when I tried to remember the questions and correct answers that I had just reviewed minutes before, my mind was confused and blank. I had never experienced this before, and it scared the hell out of me. When I returned home from work that night, I didn't mention anything about the test to Robyn. I was too embarrassed.

In addition to my confused mind, my speaking had become weak and strained. The connection between my mind and mouth wasn't working—words became lost in the transfer. Sometimes I slurred my speech when I met clients and during team meetings, and I worried that my thinking and speaking skills were adversely affecting my work.

As it turns out, my clouded mind and strained speech had not gone unnoticed. Shortly after I failed my test, my career manager, Barc, organized a speaking course and suggested I sign up when it started in

January. Barc had been with the company for three years, compared to my almost eight, so I was reluctant to follow his lead; however, we had successfully worked together on a number of projects and had always had each other's back, so I signed up for the course in hopes of arresting the downward spiral.

The final project was to give a brief five-minute speech on the topic of my choice. It didn't matter what topic I picked—the course hadn't made my speaking any more fluid or my thinking any clearer. When I spoke, I was terrible. I read word for word from my notes, rushing, terrified that I might lose my place. I didn't lift my eyes off the page to connect with listeners. I didn't follow any of the principles of effective public speaking that were reinforced during the class. When I finished, my classmates sugarcoated the truth when they constructively critiqued my performance. I imagined how uncomfortable it must have been for them to watch me flounder and trip over my words.

When I returned home that night, I had to face Robyn. I had practiced my presentation with her the three previous nights, so there was no way to avoid the subject.

"Hey Honey, how'd it go?" she asked when I entered the kitchen.

"Fine, I received good feedback. Several of my coworkers said they would replace their incandescent bulbs with compact fluorescent ones when they burned out."

I knew she wanted more details, but I hadn't made sense of what had occurred earlier in the day and could only feed her the same sugarcoated feedback. I knew this wouldn't satisfy her, but it was all I could muster.

I felt shame. I was frustrated and humiliated. Typically, I would "ride" my way out of the gloom, but it was winter in LA, rainy and cold. There was no escaping to the Santa Monica Mountains to center myself, and I was unmotivated to go to the gym. Even if I had found the desire, my body wouldn't have cooperated.

After work each day, I limped out the door and dragged myself home to sit on the couch and mindlessly watch TV. If lucky, I caught a catnap and moderately recharged. If I was obsessed about events of the day, I would fall into a television-induced coma for a few hours until it was time for bed. I had fallen into an abyss of hopelessness as my body failed me. I shuffled my feet like a ninety-five-year-old man, my hands and feet numb, my strength and balance deteriorating, my mind turning in circles. I couldn't piss standing, I was falling down stairs, failing tests, and I could barely talk.

One morning that winter, as I dressed for work, I tried to button my shirt. I grasped a button in my right hand, the good one, and tried to guide it into place with my fingers. When my fingers went to push the button through the buttonhole, they didn't work. My mind knew what it wanted to do, but my fingers didn't receive the signal. I was a prisoner in my own body. Robyn, who was in the room with me getting ready for work, saw me struggle and she finished the job.

MS was stealing my independence. We hadn't even been married a year, yet Robyn had to care for me as if I was a frail, elderly man. Though her care deepened my love for her, I knew I had to do something about my health.

Because of my trouble walking, I assumed the day I needed a walker, then a wheelchair, was near. I also assumed that my days at work were numbered. I worried if I could continue to be the husband Robyn needed and deserved. This wasn't the great life the doctor encouraged me to lead the day I learned about the diagnosis. Rather than sit idly on the sideline as I wasted away, I finally decided to take action.

I searched for stories about others who improved their MS condition. I had pursued conventional drug therapies such as Rebif,

Avonex, and Copaxone over the last two years with questionable results, so I was open to anything, even non-traditional approaches—a huge stretch for me considering my addiction to analytical thinking.

During my search, I found an inspirational story about a guy in his thirties, Matthew Grace. He had suffered significant bodily damage from the effects of MS and had adopted a raw food lifestyle. As the result of months of hard work and an unyielding commitment to the raw lifestyle, he regained use of his legs. Before his turn around, he was in a wheelchair. After several years, he recovered to the point where he could run. His story gave me hope that I might be able to improve, even reverse my condition.

After the intervention the previous fall, Pete was eager to support my efforts. In January, he planned to travel down to the Optimum Health Institute (OHI) in San Diego for a week to cleanse and set his goals for the New Year. Another reason he wanted to go was to see if the institute might help me. He felt the institute's mission to help people unify their mind, body, and spirit through food, body detoxification, and rejuvenation held promise. The institute opened its doors every Sunday to visitors. This coincided with Pete's first meal there, and he invited me to join him.

I checked out the OHI website to see what it was all about. My first impression was that it had a strong spiritual overtone, but as I read more, the healing practices seemed to be grounded in physiological and psychological thought. I found that the institute's healing philosophy was based on the healing principles of the Essene people, known for their hygiene and dietary principles. The philosophy emphasized a healing approach that enabled a person to tap their body's inherent healing mechanisms. I didn't totally get what it meant, but I liked the idea of unlocking my body's ability to heal.

Optimistic about the prospect of a recovery, I drove the two hours from Santa Monica to San Diego alone, hoping OHI held the answers I needed. Robyn didn't join me because what she read about the program led her to conclude it was too religious. At dinner, my plate was filled with tons of colors. I saw every vegetable imaginable, from purple cabbage to green sprouts to orange carrots, yellow squash and a brownish-red sea vegetable called dulse. My plate was full, but it left me less than satisfied. I craved pizza, pasta, chile relleno, or a bean and cheese burrito, my staple diet for most of my adult life.

I got through dinner because I knew I could treat myself to one of my favorite dishes when I got home. There was an introductory overview while we ate given by the director, Pam Nees, who started the program with her husband thirty years earlier and had carried on the institute's mission after his passing. Pam was in her sixties. Her long blond hair was pulled back in a ponytail and she wore no makeup and reminded me of a Sunday school teacher. Her conservative appearance ironically made me feel more comfortable about the radical program she espoused, and for some reason I listened.

I learned that OHI was founded in 1976 as a retreat center affiliated with the Free Sacred Trinity Church based on Essene dietary and hygiene practices. The principles had been taught at Hippocrates of Boston, opened by Ann Wigmore to help people regain their health naturally through live, whole food, body detoxification, and spiritual enlightenment. Over the thirty years OHI had been in operation, more than 75,000 people from around the world had visited the retreat center to improve not only their health, but also their lives.

Pam emphasized that all of our bodies are programmed to be vibrantly healthy and that if our health is failing, we all have the ability to regain it through the institute's program of body detoxification, whole, live-food dietary regimen, exercise, and mind-body-spirit unification. I sat and listened to "pious Pam" speak and grew skeptical. The place sounded too touchy-feely and New Age-y. The presentation struck me as fraudulent—the place seemed too good to be true, and nobody was really *that nice,* but I was desperate, so I continued to listen to the basics about raw food.

Raw food wasn't cooked above 118 degrees, nor was it irradiated or processed, so the food's natural enzymes remained intact, which helped the body metabolize food more efficiently. These natural enzymes were the catalyst that began the digestion process. I had never put much thought into what happened to food after I put it in my mouth. I didn't care about the details; I just wanted to satisfy my hunger.

What I heard next was the essence of the OHI healing program. I learned that digestion placed a huge metabolic load on the body that was lifted when a person ate raw plant-based foods and cleansed their colon. The energy used to digest enzyme-depleted, cooked food, was freed to help the body heal. I made the mental leap and understood why the OHI program held hope for me. Raw food meant less effort for my struggling body, and possibly resulted in more energy. I wanted to jump up and yell "I get it!" but I needed to understand what I could actually eat before I became too excited.

I was relieved to learn that raw food consisted of raw fruits, vegetables, nuts, seeds, and fermented foods like sauerkraut, which all appealed to me. Eating raw was looking like a possibility. While the raw food would be an adjustment for my taste buds and my sense of what it meant for my stomach to be full, I liked the promise it held to improve my health.

Before she closed, Pam briefly spoke about an exciting opportunity the institute offered known as the missionary program. When she said the word 'missionary' I felt my body resist. I was suspicious of any religious undertones because I didn't like any beliefs or ideals forced on me. Pam must have known about this possible reaction because she said OHI missionaries guided people on healing not religious journeys; they signed on for a minimum of three months, immersed themselves in the program, and provided eighteen hours of service per week: working in the kitchen, the garden, and leading daily exercises and welcome tours. They adhered to the live, raw organic vegan diet and detox program, participated in exercise, attended classes, and led group affirmation sessions before each meal. They focused on healing twenty-four hours per day, seven days per week. The promise of renewed health strongly resonated, and I wanted to be a missionary.

Pam concluded by repeating a characteristic of the program that hadn't stuck when she said it at the start. She reiterated that guests needed to understand that their journey to optimal health would be primarily self-guided. The program was rooted in commonly accepted scientific principles of nutrition, anatomy, and digestion, but she said guests needed to know there was no medical staff to confirm our health was improving. She said that would be self-evident, and that the confirmation would come from within.

When I got home, I had an insatiable hunger for information on raw food. I pursued every reasonable lead. I didn't have anything to lose and the more I read, the more I understood I had a lot to gain by considering this lifestyle change.

The weekend after my visit to OHI, I had a conversation with my mom that reinforced the promise of food and its ability to heal. My mom related a conversation she had had with her hairstylist earlier that afternoon. Her stylist had a client whose husband had recovered from the impacts of multiple sclerosis through a macrobiotic diet.

I realized a lifestyle shift might help me, too. The tingling that had started in my hands and feet a year and a half earlier had turned into pain on a good day, when I could feel anything at all. As I rapidly lost mental capacity at work and physical capability on the bike, I was motivated to find some way to stop the progression.

More, my continuing troubles in bed contributed to a growing feeling of hopelessness. I had to find a way out of the darkness and, if possible, reverse the damage. After talking with Robyn, my first step was to ask for a three-month leave of absence from Sapient, so I wrote a letter to the company's dual CEOs.

Dear Stu and Jerry,

It is with great excitement and enthusiasm that I write this letter. I believe I have found a place that will allow me to restore my health from the effects of MS that I have struggled with over the past eight years and which has now significantly impacted my quality of life.

My Multiple Sclerosis condition is declining. Attack episodes over the past three years have left me in a state where my balance, mobility and strength have been impacted. I am concerned that if my current state of health does not improve, I will not be able to work to my full potential in the future. Now is the time to take action to improve my health.

I am writing this letter to request a three month disability leave from Sapient to improve my health before it deteriorates further and while my health can be positively impacted with an aggressive program that I will describe later in this letter. My professional relationship with Sapient is very important to me and I want to take restorative steps that are possible now. My desire and goal is to have my future contribution to Sapient be equal to or better than it has been in the past and this leave will help to insure that.

The Optimum Health Institute (OHI) is a cutting edge program where people go to restore themselves from the impacts of health conditions like MS. Through diet, exercise, meditation and education one is able to restore their bodies. It takes a minimum of 3 months to restore oneself from a health challenge according to the institute. Optimum Health is a cutting edge health program in San Diego, which has been in existence for over 30 years. Tens of thousands of people from all over the world who face health challenges or want to avoid them have gone to OHI.

According to OHI, one must immerse themselves into a program with no outside distraction and OHI is set up for people to operate for an extended period of time in an environment where the only focus is learning how to restore the body through raw food, yoga, meditation and new modes of thinking and speaking that lead to healing. People are able to restore themselves from the impacts of health conditions such as cancer and MS. My MS Neurologist, Dr. Andrew Woo, is in favor of me participating in this program. I am really optimistic about the restorative possibilities of OHI, and I hope that Sapient will support me in this effort. After completion of the program, I want to return to Sapient.

I knew I was taking a huge chance by sending the letter that might end my career, but I was desperate. I had to find some way to improve my health, even if I had no idea if the program would work for me, or if I would even be accepted as a missionary. Robyn and I put our fate in the hands of a higher power; we made arrangements to stay at the institute for the initial three weeks.

A few days after I sent the letter, I received word that my time off had been approved. I felt a huge sense of relief knowing the company supported my decision, but I also knew the OHI program had to work and help me find my way back to health. I desperately needed to regain my independence and contribute at home and at work.

20

MOVING TOWARD OPTIMUM HEALTH

Doubts swirled in my mind as I set out on my healing journey. My research and experience lead me to conclude that care for multiple sclerosis patients usually involved making them more comfortable as they slowly wasted away; it didn't involve healing their symptoms. How could I be sure that OHI held the answer? I wondered if my first six and a half active years after the diagnosis had been a fluke. Was a wheelchair inevitable?

I had recently read about people who had improved their condition through alternative methods, but such examples weren't accepted nor promoted by allopathic ("Western") medicine. I had only anecdotal evidence; I found no medical research to support my decision to attend OHI and began to wonder if reality had finally caught up to me. I wanted to see evidence that I could fight the slow onset of paralysis. I had no idea that I would soon rely on myself to prove that someone could improve their symptoms.

On Sunday, April 10, 2005, Robyn and I stood holding hands in the courtyard waiting for the missionary to begin our welcome tour at OHI. I made a pledge to myself to fully commit to the program to see if it would improve my condition and had left Copaxone and Lipitor, the two prescription drugs I was taking, at home. I consulted with Andy before going to OHI. He was in favor of me changing my lifestyle to improve my health, but he didn't recommend I stop taking the Copaxone. I was on my own on that.

◆

As we walked the institute grounds, I struggled to keep up with the group. My lack of balance caused me to lunge for light poles, clutch handrails, and take stairs slowly. I descended the back stairs by the wheatgrass greenhouse, and my legs nearly gave out. I reached the bottom and stopped to rest. I leaned on Robyn to steady myself. After just a few minutes of motion, I suffered from vertigo. I felt like a top that had spun out of control. My body was weak. When I did conjure the strength and nerve to walk, I wasn't always confident my legs would carry me.

I kept the pace of an elderly man. From my knees to the bottom of my feet, I completely lacked feeling. It was like walking through thick, soft sand with each step. On the tour, I took short eight-inch steps. I had lost the ability to judge distances. When we finally reached the garden, I took a seat in a chair that looked conspicuously out of place. A guest must have taken it from the meeting room at the top of the hill. I was grateful to sit, because I had reached my limit.

I sat and considered my decision to attend OHI. I had just stepped away from the outside world and would be there a month. If I was accepted as a missionary, I would stay three more months. In the quiet stillness of the garden, my mind raced.

What had I done?

I had a great job, lived in a nice house, in a great neighborhood, and I had just married a wonderful woman. I had created the great life that I once imagined, but that vision was an illusion. My body didn't thrive in the environment required to support the lifestyle I had chosen, but if I didn't have my health, nothing else mattered.

The group walked to the back of the garden, and I slowly stood to follow. The path snaked its way through healthy well-tended vegetable beds. It was early spring, so the recently planted seedlings of cucumber, zucchini, tomatoes, and corn were just taking root in the nutrient-rich soil. The trail probably appeared flat to most guests, but I found it treacherous. Each bump or rock threw me off balance.

I was relieved when we finally climbed the brick steps out of the garden and stood on the evenly graded pavement of the parking lot. We walked upstairs to the multipurpose room and waited for the orientation. After Pam delivered the overview, Robyn and I grabbed dinner, piling our plates high with an assortment of sprouts and vegetables. I remembered the meal from a few months earlier during my visit with Pete, but Robyn wasn't prepared for what we'd been served.

"Is this it?" she asked.

That was the extent of her protest, but I could tell by her body language and the look on her face that she wasn't pleased. While we ate, we met a number of our fellow first-weekers, including a guy, Fabritzio, who would become my buddy. I didn't ask why he was there, because I wanted to adhere to the institute guideline of not discussing our health "opportunities" (vs. conditions), but I could tell from the bulging vein in his left arm that his health suffered—an indication of dialysis. I learned he planned to stay for the three-week program like me and hoped to continue the lifestyle on his own at home.

I cleaned my plate and looked over at Robyn. I gave her a grin of gratitude for her support. Then I looked at her plate and was overcome with concern. She had barely touched her meal.

"Everything alright? You haven't eaten much," I said.

"Yeah, I'm okay. I'm not really hungry."

It worried me that Robyn hadn't eaten dinner because I knew the cupboards back at our place were bare, so she wouldn't get anything more to eat before we went to bed, but I let it go. I knew she could take care of herself. We finished dinner and walked down the hill to our townhouse. We were both really tired and didn't have a television, so we went straight to bed.

"Good night, babe. Thanks again for agreeing to come down here," I said as I got into bed.

"The people are so friendly and supportive, but I'm hungry," she said, not holding back. "The food didn't taste good, but I wish I had gulped it down anyway."

I nodded, feeling guilty for denying her a pleasurable meal, hoping she would eat the next day—if the menu could ever tempt her to bite into the raw truth with me.

♦

The next morning I woke, juiced my morning dose of wheatgrass, and then attended exercise. As class ended, I lay on the floor with my eyes shut. The hour-long workout gave me a true sense of how much my body had deteriorated. At one point, when I bent over to stretch my back, I saw that many guests could touch their toes. I could only extend my fingers to just above my knees. When I used to stretch before a ride or run, I would routinely place my palm on the ground past my feet, but that was a distant memory.

I didn't have the flexibility, leg strength, or balance to complete many of the exercises. When the time came to walk around the compound, we were supposed to take two laps, the equivalent of a mile, but I had to stop after one. I was too fatigued to go around a second time. My one lap wasn't even a full one. I had to cut out the walk around the pool. The path seemed too narrow to navigate without tripping and falling, and I didn't want to slow everyone else behind me—that was not the first impression I wanted to make, so I turned around and headed back up the hill. It was hard to believe I had ever run a marathon or biked up any mountain, let alone ever walked a mile.

The next two days at OHI were a blur. We woke each day at 6:30 to be at exercise by 7:30, with two ounces of freshly juiced wheatgrass to cleanse our systems. Robyn and I attended seven hours of classroom lecture, learning how the digestive system works and how it holds half the body's immune system. I understood the reason for daily enemas and why the institute put such a focus on helping me and others get our digestive and elimination systems running properly.

Each day, I drank sixty-four ounces of water to adequately hydrate my body and drank four ounces of wheatgrass juice to cleanse my circulatory system and provide my body with a spectrum of vitamins, minerals, and enzymes. I also consumed thirty-two ounces of a fermented sour drink called rejuvelac to re-colonize my colon with healthy bacteria after daily colon irrigations that "steam cleaned" my insides.

I was also encouraged to begin spiritual exploration and heard about the role emotions played in healing, but I didn't do much about either. It was all I could do to keep up with the program's physical demands. Besides, I was at a total loss for what spiritual exploration meant and had no idea how to begin to understand the role my emotions played in my healing. I believed that facing my feelings was a waste of time and had the potential to sidetrack my healing—though I decided to keep an open mind.

At the end of each day, my mind was still clouded; it spun in overdrive trying to make sense of all the new information. Overwhelmed, my head hit the pillow at 10:30 each night. I would crash hard until I woke at 6:30 the next day to do it all over again committed to doing everything reasonably possible to improve my condition.

◆

On the morning of my third day, after exercise, I laid on the floor in child's pose and scanned my body. I was hungry, my head ached, and my energy was low. The detox was in full swing. I craved something sweet and would have done anything to substitute my morning wheatgrass for a can of Red Bull.

I hadn't had contact with the outside world for three days. We didn't have a television in our apartment, cell phones were instructed to be turned off, and newspapers weren't available in the reading room. I took the opportunity to step away from my old routine, but I yearned for comfort food and information that represented my old existence and gave me a sense of being normal. Because of the advancing symptoms of MS, I felt I had a gun to my head. The promise of renewed health was a powerful force that kept me on track while I adapted to what I would later call my *new normal*.

As exercise ended, I saw Robyn in the middle of the room and limped toward her.

"Hey Babe, how you feeling?" I said as I hugged her.

"The bed sucks, I'm hungry, and it feels like someone cracked me over the head with a frying pan."

"I'm sorry. It's probably the detox. We'll be at breakfast soon," I said.

"I know it's the detox, but that doesn't change how I feel. I'm tired, and if one more person tells me, 'It's part of the process,' I'm going to scream. I want more than juiced cucumber, celery, and zucchini."

Though I didn't like to hear Robyn struggle, I appreciated her ability to express her emotions. The program was kicking my ass, too. As I began to detox from my sugar, caffeine, and refined wheat diet, my body was confused. I wanted to tell her I was struggling as well but didn't, because I wanted to appear strong. I also didn't want to express any degree of my frustration, fearful it might cause us to walk away.

It was circle time, and I stood shoulder to shoulder with the other guests, dressed in a wool cap, a heavy sweatshirt, and loose mountaineering pants. The woman to my left gently took my hand, and drew me into the warm, welcoming OHI cocoon. I reluctantly looked toward her, smiled and said, "Good morning."

Morning circle was part of the OHI program intended to fill our minds with healthy uplifting thoughts. The rationale for the daily kickoff was based on the work of Deepak Chopra, who found that the mind had roughly sixty thousand thoughts daily—fewer than 5% were new. The remaining 95% were recycled thoughts and beliefs. If those thoughts and beliefs supported your life vision, then great, they could stay. If they didn't support your vision, then they needed to change. I had an opportunity at OHI to change my beliefs, nurture healing thoughts, and improve my condition. The importance of my mind's role in my healing was clear.

Once all the guests were in a circle, the program facilitator, Kimberly, gave a brief overview of the day's activities, and explained our breakfast options: vegetable or watermelon juice. I wanted to groan. This menu was not exactly the hearty egg and cheese bagel, I craved, but I chose the all-vegetable juice, even though it was the more extreme option for my tastes. I didn't want to stress my nervous system and wanted to limit my sugar intake as much as possible in support of my healing.

Kimberly asked a volunteer to come up and pull the word of the day out of a jar. A woman stepped forward, grabbed a piece of paper from the jar, and read the word perseverance. Kimberly gave the definition, emphasizing how challenging circumstances presented the opportunity to persevere. She reminded us that when faced with challenge it was important to keep our goal in mind and follow the path toward our goal even if it meant having to endure discomfort; it was through finding harmony in the midst of chaos that we were able to grow, evolve, and transcend our challenge.

I looked at Robyn and gave her a nod. She smiled as Kimberly reiterated the importance of managing our thoughts to aid healing.

I liked Kimberly. She had a spiritual, grounded way about her. She had taught a class earlier in the week called Mental Detox and knew a lot about using the mind to heal. She said it was important to have only positive, health-affirming thoughts circulating and introduced the "cancel-cancel tool" to banish unwanted words. She suggested we repeat "cancel-cancel" when a negative thought popped in our heads until our mind changed the channel. It sounded hokey, but I did it anyway, even though I was tired of "circle time" and wanted to yell, "Come on already; let's eat!" (or in our case, drink!). By the morning of the third day, I was hungry and exhausted and just wanted to be left alone.

Kimberly ended by reading from *God Spoke to Me*, a book of inspirational verses that ask the reader to have total faith in the process of living—to trust God, the universe, spirit, love—however one referred to a divine source. The passages affirmed an inherent wisdom and intelligence in everything, which could be contacted by turning within.

Kimberly confirmed that each of us could hear God's voice if we tried. I believed in God—my mother was Catholic, but I was skeptical of the idea of putting the outcome I needed, renewed health, in his hands. Ever since that cold fall night behind the woodpile, I was reluctant to put my faith in anyone's hands but my own. Since I had married Robyn, my drive to do things alone had softened, so I remained open to the idea.

Before the circle broke, Kimberly reminded us that Wednesday before lunch was an important time at the institute—the burning ceremony. She asked us to bring the scraps of paper we had collected since the start of the week, on which we had written beliefs we wanted to banish forever. We would burn our unwanted words and would replace the cast-out notions with ones that supported our vibrant life visions.

The talk about retraining my mind left me with the impression that I might have walked into a New Age cult. After all, San Diego was the home of Heaven's Gate, the sneaker-clad UFO-worshiping youth, who had made the news during my grad school days, so I vigilantly watched and listened, wary of the Kool-Aid.

That afternoon, I found myself in a circle on the front lawn of the institute, standing with a dozen or so guests ready to banish my word "perfectionism." Though I had been at OHI for only three days, I already recognized that my drive for perfection had not served me well. While I had accomplished a lot, I'd lost connection with myself.

My earliest memory of seeking perfection was as a little boy in first grade. I was seated at my desk, completing a mathematics worksheet. I had to be the first kid to turn in my work; I felt like my life depended on it. I jumped up when finished, raced a classmate to the front of the room, and slammed my worksheet in the basket.

It was like I had a hand in the middle of my back that pushed me forward—to be first, to be best, to be perfect. The pressure never let up. I wasn't comfortable unless I did something in pursuit of perfection. When I did reach a goal at work, school, or after a race, I didn't allow myself to relax but, instead, I searched for my next ambition, as if the only way I could love myself was by achieving more. In that case, why wait, right? Though I didn't have all the answers that afternoon, it seemed that part of the reason my health was failing was due to my refusal to pause and reflect on what this drive for perfection was really doing to my body. But that was about to change.

I pulled out the scrap of paper and threw it in the fire, searching for a new word to replace the word "perfection," as suggested by the woman facilitating this exercise. She told us that when you banish a thought, you need to replace it with a new idea to fill the empty space. If I didn't choose a thought to fill the void, then my mind would indiscriminately find some random thought or belief to fill it. That scared me. I couldn't trust my mind to serve my healing interests. Since the diagnosis, that hadn't worked too well. I had achieved a lot but lost my health. Instead of perfection, I chose the word self-acceptance; I could love myself, and I was good enough without my achievements. It sounded good. I just wondered how the simple belief might serve my well being. I decided to suspend judgment and see where the change might lead.

The facilitator asked one last time if there was anything else anyone wanted to give away. I looked down at the red rubber MS bracelet on my wrist that Robyn had given me. I leaned over and whispered in her ear.

"I know you gave this to me as a show of support, but I want to give it away. It's a constant reminder of the impact the MS has on me. You mind if I throw it in?"

"Go for it, and you can have mine while you're at it."

I reached down, slid the band off my wrist. Robyn handed me hers, and we threw them into the fire. The facilitator ended the session, and I squeezed Robyn's hand, feeling a heavy burden lift from my shoulders. I was not drinking the Kool-Aid. If anything, I had stopped drinking my own.

By the end of my first week, I knew the program held promise. The raw food, wheatgrass shots and enemas, new thinking, yoga, and exercise had already positively affected my body. I felt strength return to my legs and noticed feeling returning to my fingers. They tingled and burned, and though it was unpleasant, it was better than feeling nothing at all.

21

SERIOUSLY? A CONVERSATION WITH MS

My journey into mind-body connection continued. I never considered that my "condition" held a message until I attended a Mind-Body Connection class facilitated by Dr. Bob Price, who held a Ph.D. in psychology. The notion seemed absurd on the surface. *You mean MS is trying to talk to me?* My analytical mind was freaking out. How could this be? Who was this guy that fiercely defended his premise: the key to healing was to listen to the message inside whatever was ailing us— cancer, arthritis, unhappiness, or any other physical or emotional illness a person faced?

I needed to listen to Dr. Bob, despite my reservations. He was a slight man in his late seventies with an engaging style. He had served the Los Angeles Fire Department twenty years earlier. I wasn't sure how a retired LA firefighter was qualified to help me heal, so I almost tuned him out, until he said he had spent two days per week counseling cancer patients and his free time studying for his degree in psychology.

After he retired from the fire department, he received his doctorate in psychology and focused on counseling cancer patients until the spark ran out. He had been having the same conversations week after week with the same people without much progress. One day he came up with a simple healing concept known as the "Price Parts Model" to help people recover—based on his experience fighting fires.

In the case of healing, Dr. Bob's approach helped people identify the unwanted condition, reject it, and start to heal, the key being to listen to any message held within that condition. For this communication to happen, the patient had to sit and listen to what the condition (illness, unwanted belief system, etc.) had to say and then do what it suggested. The problem would back off and would be resolved accordingly.

It was a lot to take in. Dr. Bob contended that all illnesses or conditions were psychosomatic unless proven otherwise, and if proven otherwise, the mind still played a significant role in their existence. I had heard enough. I wanted to jump up, hop on stage, and wring his scrawny neck. There was no way the pain and stiffness that plagued me weren't real. I looked around, caught my buddy Fabritzio's attention, and rolled my eyes.

If the class hadn't been required to receive a "raw" certification and become eligible to apply to be a missionary, I would have left, but I couldn't. Early experience had proven that the OHI program improved my symptoms, so I sucked it up and stayed.

I wouldn't exactly say I was having a breakthrough in this class—not yet at least, but my mind was definitely being broken open, whether I liked it or not. Dr. Bob's theory satisfied my rational mind and, apparently, his theory had scientific backing. Albert Einstein had alluded to the same: "We can't solve problems by using the same kind of thinking as when we created them." According to Dr. Bob, we are all controlled by our thinking—*energy follows intention,* and the Parts Model allowed a person to use their mind to make a conscious decision to improve their health; simple enough.

Dr. Bob illustrated the model in action, asking if anyone in the audience intended to change something about their life—inevitably, a bunch of hands went up. Then he asked who wanted to change something right now. A few brave souls kept their hands raised. He focused on a middle-aged woman in the front row and looked her in the eye.

"You want to change something, well let's get to it."

The woman walked to the front and sat in one of the two empty chairs. He asked her name. "Judy," she said.

"So, Judy, what do you want to change?"

"I have this voice in my head that always tells me I'm not good enough."

"How long have you heard that voice?"

"Since I was a girl."

"So it's been around for a while and you want to get rid of it?"

"Yes."

"When?"

"Now would be good."

"Okay, so what do you want to say to the voice?"

"Go away."

"No, don't look at me, say it to the voice. Its right there," he said pointing to the empty chair.

"Voice, go away. I want you gone."

"Okay, now stand up and switch chairs."

It was funny to watch her get up and change seats to continue a conversation with an invisible part of herself. I heard a few muted, nervous chuckles as she stood. She now sat in the same chair as her judgmental voice, and Dr. Bob asked her voice to respond.

"No," Judy's rational voice shot back. "It's not that easy."

Dr. Bob asked, "What do you need to leave Judy alone?"

"I need her to quit being so hard on herself and to see herself as a good person who does the best she can."

It was clear from her response that Judy had probably asked the voice to leave her alone before, but probably hadn't used the Parts Model to engage it in conversation, or it might not have been around. Dr. Bob asked Judy to stand up and change seats. The honesty of Judy's conversation was apparent by the silenced room.

"What do you think?" Dr. Bob asked as Judy sat.

"I think I can do that," she said as her voice cracked.

"Do what?" he said.

"Back off myself and see what I do as good enough."

Dr. Bob said that changes can occur after just one conversation, but that it was often best to have follow-up conversations with yourself to be sure the change held. "Judy, can you agree to meet once a week to make sure the voice doesn't return?"

"Yes, I can," she said.

When class ended, I remained in my seat. There was no way a conversation with the MS would help me heal. It seemed way too easy and more than a little odd. Popular culture led me to believe I would never be able to heal, at least not fully. MS was a complex disease. The medical community didn't even know what caused it.

To hear that the answer may in part lie in facing the demon of MS itself, in a chair no less, seemed disingenuous, but I was desperate to add this into my regimen, knowing the diet, detox, exercise, and new thinking already had shifted my perception about what it meant to live with MS. Though the institute discouraged guests from meeting with facilitators outside class, I received permission to meet with Dr. Bob at the end of my second week. It dawned on me that the mountain wasn't whispering my fate on Shasta, the voice I had heard was MS telling me it was time to change.

I showed up at my appointment with Dr. Bob and told him I was interested to see if the Parts Model might help me heal from MS. He invited me to have a conversation with the MS and pulled over a chair. I couldn't help but think that of all the things I had done in my life, this was one of the strangest. *I'm about to talk to my MS, unrehearsed.* I felt more than slightly out of control.

"What would you like to say to the MS?" he asked.

I stared at the empty chair, feeling foolish, trying to find a way to speak.

"I want to heal from the impacts that you have caused. What do I need to do?" While it was very weird to imagine the MS seated there next to me, I saw myself as strong, healthy, and listened intently to hear what it had to say.

"Okay, now stand up and switch chairs," Dr. Bob instructed.

I stood, feeling self-conscious. I was relieved that only Dr. Bob was watching.

Dr. Bob said, "Go ahead. What do you think about what Jon just asked you?"

I took a deep breath and felt my body relax. "You know if you want to heal, you need to back off yourself and not try so hard to be perfect."

There was no hesitation. The words rushed through me. I might have unlocked their cage during the burning ceremony my first week as a guest, but it was clear I still had more work to release the limiting belief.

"Now switch chairs," Dr. Bob instructed.

I got up and moved to my original seat. I sat and hesitated for a few seconds.

"Is there anything else you want to ask the MS?" Dr. Bob said.

"Is this all I need to do to heal?" I asked.

I got up and switched seats.

"It's a start, but let's keep talking and meeting twice a week just like this."

I got up and switched chairs. I looked over at Dr. Bob. "Is that it?" I asked.

"Looks like it. Are you going to be able to do this on your own?"

"I will. I'm here to heal and will make the time."

I remained seated and was amazed at the simplicity of our interaction. It seemed too easy. I figured I would need to have several more conversations to hear more about what I needed to do to heal, but I was eager to integrate the Parts Model into my routine. There was something liberating about the whole experience. I realized there was no me and you with the MS. We were one and the same; it was time to end the duality. I had been fighting something that I should be integrating.

Dr. Bob was a trained hypnotherapist and asked if there were any incidents that I might have held from my past that I wanted to let go of in order to accelerate my healing. I sat quietly with the question, and I looked around his office. My gaze settled on a pair of native African-looking statues on his bookshelf. Then it came to me. The incident when I was a scared kid, a five-year-old boy crying behind the woodpile.

I told him all about that night, and he asked if I wanted to go through a guided meditation to eliminate the emotional charge and help my mind and body heal. I eagerly agreed. I was up for anything that might heal this wound.

"Let's go back to that night. Tell me all about where you are and how you're feeling," Dr. Bob began.

"I'm standing alone behind the woodpile. It's cold, so I'm shivering, and my head is buried in my arms."

"What else?" he asked.

"I'm a little boy, and I'm scared. I'm crying. I think something may have happened to my mom."

"What may have happened to your mom?"

"I'm scared she may have been shot and killed by the Mafia."

"What else do you feel?"

"I feel like I am responsible for keeping myself safe."

"What else. Do you feel anything else?"

"I feel alone."

"Anything else?"

"That's it."

Doctor Bob then guided me through a meditation session to take away the emotional charge of being alone by the woodpile. He guided me through a meditation where my mom held me in her arms like an infant and made me feel safe. Something was shifting in me. I was starting to let go of the things that didn't serve me.

♦

I embraced the OHI ritual: I began each day with inspirational thoughts, drank the required amounts of water, wheatgrass, and rejuvelac, fasted and juiced Monday through Thursday afternoon, ate fresh, raw food at each meal Thursday night through Sunday, did daily colon irrigations, purged unwanted beliefs and replaced them with positive, health affirming concepts, attended every class, and even had a few conversations with MS.

I mindfully moved through each day implementing the program and giving it every opportunity to work. None of the tools I adopted, on their own, were difficult to use, but taken together, they represented a major lifestyle shift. After three weeks, filled with fifteen-hour days of healing activity, I noticed my condition changing.

I felt the physical changes first—my balance, endurance, and strength improved. I started to walk around the pool during morning exercise, which was significant because for the first two weeks, the path felt too narrow to navigate without falling. By the third week, I routinely made it twice around the grounds on the walk. The changes ran deeper than physical. I had developed a vision for my healing journey—to heal from the damage MS had inflicted on my body, to speak fluidly, think clearly, and walk easily.

My old philosophy—one that pushed me to every limit, had run its course. As I regained feeling and function after the onset of paralysis, I realized the importance of the mind, body, and spirit triad to heal. I realized I was not destined to a life of increased paralysis, but rather that my body was programmed to return to its original state of optimal health if I filled it with the right food, liquids, and thoughts. The biggest shift was to accept MS into my heart, to treat it as my coach, and to ask it for guidance in my healing journey. Though I had lost eighteen pounds, going from 167 to 149, my hope had been renewed.

On Friday morning of my third week, I received my diploma, and by noon I had turned in my application for the missionary program. The following week I stayed at the institute alone while Robyn traveled back east to celebrate her nephew's first birthday. Tuesday of that week, I received news I was accepted as a missionary.

22

THE HEALING GARDEN

Before I started my post as a missionary, I spent a week at home. I meditated daily, visited a local health food store twice a day for doses of fresh wheatgrass juice, drank homemade rejuvelac, and ate only raw food. I even tried a few enemas. Not exactly a homecoming party festivity, but helpful. I remained fully committed to the program, at least the parts I understood well enough to incorporate.

The first thing I did on Monday morning at home was call Sapient to give them an update on my condition and ask for an additional month of leave to complete the missionary program. I had been granted three months of leave but would need four to complete my missionary commitment. The human resources executive I spoke with was impressed with my progress. She listened to my update but didn't immediately grant my request. She told me she would get back to me with a decision after she received approval. I wasn't sure how I would handle things if my request was denied.

Instead of worry, I spent time looking for three pieces of exercise equipment that I had heard about during my initial stay—a mini-trampoline, leg weights, and a Reebok TIS board. They were supposed to help me continue to rebuild my strength and regain my balance. I found each and hoped to integrate them into my daily routine.

Based on my time as a guest, I knew my days would be full between my work in the garden and my healing activities, but I wanted to make the most of my opportunity.

While at home, I stayed on the diet through willpower and Robyn's help. She saw my improvement and wanted to support my continued healing. She was trying to eat 100% raw for me, to better understand what I was going through, and because she liked how clean and light eating raw made her feel—even after all that initial complaining. She even signed up for raw food classes taught by noted raw chefs in LA to learn what she needed to make sure I had raw food for breakfast, lunch, and dinner—and I miraculously resisted a visit to Holy Guacamole, my favorite Mexican joint, during my week at home.

"How'd it go?" I asked when Robyn returned from her first raw food class.

"Awesome. We made this really yummy tomato soup and a walnut nut loaf and I learned how to dehydrate crackers."

"Sounds so good, I can't wait to try them."

"It's funny. I enjoy making raw food; it reminds me of learning to make vegetable sushi rolls with my parent's friend Mitsue when I was a girl."

Hearing her talk, I was reminded again how lucky I was to have her as my wife. I imagined her as this resourceful girl. She probably had had a picture of another life rather than one toughing it out by the side of a husband with MS, but it seemed she was going to make the best of it and work with me to turn things around.

Though it felt good to reconnect with Robyn, I worried about our separation while I was at OHI. I knew it was a lot to ask of my new bride to be okay with my three-month absence, but we were both fueled by the hope that the raw food and detox program would help me find my way back to a great life. Though concerns lingered about what might happen to us if I didn't regain my health, I tried not to engage them when they surfaced. I would use the cancel-cancel tool to banish anything negative from my consciousness.

Despite any reservations I had about threatening our relationship, I knew I had a lot deeper to go into alternative healing. When concerns surfaced, I focused on the handful of people who improved their MS conditions there; I wanted to be one of them.

My gut told me that I was healing. I had learned that the body was naturally driven to heal and that food was medicine. These concepts cycled through my mind and confirmed I was on the right track, so there was no looking back. I just needed to keep the faith and supply my body with the right stuff: food, water, thoughts, and air, so I could find my way back to health.

By the end of my week at home, I received a call from Sapient. They granted my request. I continued to make final preparations for my return to OHI and packed only one bag of clothes. I could do laundry on-site. I also brought a journal with me to explore my feelings and to record the changes I was experiencing. I wanted to remember what it felt like to regain feelings and functions I had lost.

The only non-essential thing I brought was my bike. I looked forward to a ride when I regained my strength, balance, and endurance. I was optimistic in every way. Even Pam made it easier, agreeing to allow me to return home on the weekends to maintain my relationship with Robyn. Like the Texas project, I was re-learning the importance of asking for what I needed. So far, it had been easy.

I said goodbye to Robyn and returned to OHI, approaching my healing mission with a fresh perspective, on the lookout for things I had missed or didn't fully embrace the first time. On my third day back, as I sat in a class called Emotional Detox, I realized that there was an important fourth leg to the OHI program that I hadn't integrated into my healing—emotions: the real kind, the ones you dig down deep in your soul for.

It hit me that anger, resentment, and sorrow could get stuck in the body and impact health—specifically, the immune system. I understood stuck feelings were like trapped free radicals and damaged the body. During the class, I learned that our bodies could hold on to feelings that weren't effectively processed for days, months, even years.

Woah, I thought. This was huge and I wondered just how much my body had been carrying around. Since I was a boy, I was taught to avoid negative feelings at all costs and never felt comfortable talking about my feelings. As an adult, I was blinded by my drive to succeed. I had pushed my mind and body hard over the previous eight years, with insanely long work hours and misdirected beliefs about health and feelings, which had all conspired to throw me out of balance. Before OHI, I was a nervous automaton stuck in the 'on' position without time for feelings. Consequently, my health nose-dived.

It wasn't the first time I had heard about the connection between health and emotions, but it finally touched a nerve. I had almost completely overlooked my feelings during my first four weeks, just like the previous thirty years. The guided meditation I had done with Dr. Bob to deal with the emotional charge of the woodpile incident was the extent of my emotional processing as a guest. I began to suspect that my whole take on my return to health did not mean just *an absence of disease*. How about an absence of all the false beliefs and negative thoughts that had looped in my mind for years?

I had started my missionary experience committed to putting my faith in the OHI process, hoping my condition would continue to improve, and finally ready to deal with the fact that I needed to explore my negative feelings—beyond the woodpile, that had remained locked away since childhood and consequently compromised my health.

One morning, near the end of my first week back, I woke up very stiff. I thought at first the soreness was because of the bed, but then I remembered my dream. I was at work and had fallen into my old habits, and my health suffered. I was concerned that the feeling I experienced in my dream somehow became stuck in my body and had contributed to the stiffness in my back, shoulders, and legs. I had never heard of emotions being transferred from the sub-conscious to the conscious self, but it made sense.

Rather than avoid the insight and blindly go through my day, I decided to use the tool I had just learned to move the emotion through my body. I stayed in bed and went through Kimberly's six-step emotional detox process. I named the emotion, observed the feeling it created in my body, wrote about it in my journal, set an intention to release it as I worked in the garden, and planned to share my feelings with Robyn when we spoke that night. Finally, I made a note to celebrate my accomplishment several times that day—before each meal, while I worked in the garden, and during yoga.

Later that morning, I worked in the garden—watering, weeding, and picking vegetables. The work pushed me at times, but the majority was spent in an altered state of consciousness, meditating and humming, which felt healing. My life slowed down while I tended to the vegetables and looked after my own needs. That was my new routine for as long as four hours per day, five days per week.

Balance was my focus during Toning Class on Wednesday nights. I learned to hum into each of my body's seven chakras to align my body's eight spiritual centers. As the result of sitting through the class for the previous six weeks, I had realized that my life before OHI—the break-neck pace, improper diet, obsessed thoughts, and unprocessed emotions all contributed to my body going out of tune and my health declining. I welcomed the disappearance of that old, diseased existence and was excited about the new healthy, vital image of myself.

I sat in the fifty-person group and hummed the sound of each chakra for five minutes. The experience was very much like a group chanting "om" in a yoga class, except the chanting lasted forty minutes rather than a few seconds. I sat immersed in the healing sounds while each chakra became balanced. I sat through the experience a few times as a skeptic before I lowered my guard and fully opened myself up to the benefits. After several sessions, I felt balanced enough to run down the hill back to my apartment. I finally understood the merits of this "alternative" healing technique. It was the first time I had run in close to two years and was a very clear indication of my improved health.

At the end of my first week as a missionary, my body and mind continued to move away from paralysis. My body grew stronger, my endurance and equilibrium improved, feeling returned to my arms and legs, my voice became more relaxed, and my mind grasped concepts more quickly. I often thought about Robyn and wanted to impress her with my progress, but I needed to identify more areas where I could focus my attention before we spoke. A brief summary wouldn't do. She would want details.

One morning, during my second week back, as I stood and watered plants, I turned my head from side to side, seeing the thriving plants. My chin stopped at forty-five degrees rather than ninety. I was surprised. I had lost range of motion in my neck and noticed there was a sharp pain when my neck was extended at the forty-five-degree point. I also felt a strange sense of vertigo as I turned my head. The pain that resulted wasn't new; it had become a constant annoyance. I wanted to stop the hurt, improve the range of motion, and end the feelings of dizziness and imbalance.

With my eyes closed, I violently shook my head from right to left and listened. This wasn't anything I had read about. The headshakes were something I stumbled on in the moment listening to MS. They felt good, so I did them. I did twenty headshakes to each side. Having my eyes shut helped stop the feeling of vertigo. When I stopped the shakes, I kept my eyes closed and counted to sixty. The feeling of disequilibrium dissipated, and a feeling of warm contentment replaced it. I opened my eyes and concluded that my new exercise might improve my condition and decided to do head shakes three times a day for the next two weeks. I assumed it would be best to do them in private, imagining they probably seemed odd to others and not wanting to draw unnecessary attention to myself. I had found an additional area to focus my efforts that might yield a real noticeable improvement. Robyn would be impressed.

That night, after dinner, I weighed myself on my way out of the dining room. I was 136 pounds—way too thin for my five-foot, ten-inch frame. Though many guests had come to OHI specifically to lose weight, I wasn't one of them. "Damn," I said under my breath as my heart sank. I was still shedding pounds two weeks into my mission. I had most likely lost the critical muscle mass that I needed to work in the garden, to balance my body when I carried groceries, and to push open heavy doors as I moved through my day.

At 136 pounds, I weighed nearly the same as I did after my junior year in high school as a seventeen-year-old boy. The most I had ever weighed was 200 pounds, two years after I graduated from my gluttonous college days and a year and a half after being on the road eating a steady diet of pizza, fries, and hamburgers. I had dropped to 155 pounds at the height of my marathon days. I was almost twenty pounds under my lowest weight as a grown man, and it terrified me. Where was the floor? How long would this continue before I wasted away? How would I ever explain this was 'progress' to Robyn?

The OHI program was designed for people to detoxify their body and lose weight. It obviously worked for me, even if weight loss was not my intention. I wanted to continue to heal, but I needed my weight to stabilize and decided to eat a second plate of food at lunch to see if that provided the calories I needed to stop the weight loss.

One day after working in the garden, I walked up to the dining room for lunch. It was a beautiful warm sunny afternoon, so I decided to eat my lunch outside on the front lawn. When I finished, I sunk into my chair, hands relaxed, legs outstretched, feeling the warm rays. I felt some feeling return to my hands. It was a tingling, thawing sensation, similar to how I felt when I came inside following an afternoon playing in the snow in Vermont as a kid—cold needles pricking my skin through wool gloves.

As I felt the sun penetrate my body to the bone, the tingling diminished. I became curious to see what might happen if I placed my hands on the warm pavement. I got up from my chair, sat on the grass, and put my fingers on the cement. I felt the heat radiate off the concrete and penetrate my hands. The heat was so intense that it overrode the tingling. I could only stand the intensity for a few minutes, but I relished the relief from the needles, so I waited as long as I could before I lifted my hands.

I returned to my apartment that night and called Robyn. I couldn't wait to tell her about my experiment, but when I finished, she only asked, "Did anyone see you?"

I paused, sensing the accusation in her voice. I wanted to hear joy.

"I'm not sure, why?" I asked.

"I imagine you sitting on the grass with your big man hands resting on the sidewalk might have caused people to wonder about your mental stability."

"I didn't think about that, I just reacted in the moment."

Robyn didn't usually care about what others thought except when she felt really uneasy, which didn't happen very often. This was one of those times. It didn't seem like a big deal to me, but it was to her. My drive to regain my health had led me to completely look past social norms— they were the furthest thing from my mind, but Robyn had had enough of me pushing the boundaries and yearned for a sense of normalcy.

"Why can't you just be comfortable that you are in a good place with your healing and stop looking for the next thing?" she asked.

"I can't help it. Things are just coming to me in the moment."

"I worry that you're pushing yourself too hard to heal."

"I hear you," I said, feeling defensive and a little put off. "But I'm just going with the flow and doing things that feel right in the moment."

What felt right then was saying goodnight and hanging up the phone. For the first time since I'd begun the missionary program, I worried my marriage might not survive it.

On Friday of my third missionary week, I finished my work in the garden, ate lunch, packed my bag, and took a cab to the train station for my trip home. I was eager to see Robyn. Though we had talked every day, sometimes two or three times, a phone call wasn't the same as seeing her in person. Despite the intensity of our last conversation, I was still excited to see her.

When I stepped off the platform in Los Angeles, our eyes met. "Babe!" I yelled and dropped my bag and engulfed her in a hug. I drew her close but felt resistance. I realized it had been three weeks since we had seen each other and assumed she might need some time to adjust.

"I'm so happy to see you, you look great." I said, hoping she recognized the change in my condition and would respond in kind.

"I'm so happy you're home," she said with concern on her face.

All I could think was, *Is that all?* Robyn was usually effusive in her greetings. Her lack of emotion after our three-week separation alerted me that something was very wrong. As we walked to her car, we caught up. I reiterated how happy I was to see her and told her about my morning in the garden. I didn't sense she shared my excitement. As we drove down the freeway toward Santa Monica, there was very little conversation.

My mind jumped to all kinds of conclusions. Had I done something somehow to embarrass her? Had she done something to fill the void created by my three-week absence, like find comfort in the companionship of another guy? When I couldn't bare the silence any longer, I confronted her.

"What's up?"

My question was like a lightning bolt. She erupted into a storm of emotions as tears gushed down her face. She could barely speak. She was like a three-year-old who tried to talk through tears after crashing on a bike.

"I'm so scared . . . You've lost so much weight. What happened?"

I paused. Robyn had always been my mirror, and I didn't expect her reaction.

"It's the program. I'm tearing down my body, so I can rebuild it."

"I understand, but you can't go back until we figure out how to stop the weight loss. I don't know what we're going to do!"

Robyn would share later how terrified she had been that night. When she first saw me in the train station, she told me it had taken all of her strength not to break down, because I was so gaunt and thin.

Her greeting wasn't what I had expected or hoped. I had opened up to MS and had continued to improve; however, since we hadn't experienced the changes together, Robyn had been left out of the loop. All she could see was skin and bones.

"When I get back to OHI, I'll meet with Pam and make sure she passes a note to the kitchen so I can get extra food at every meal."

"I don't know if you should go back," she said.

I knew I had my work cut out for me over the next few days to bring Robyn up to speed on the changes and to make sure I was on the train back to San Diego that Sunday night—no matter how traumatic it might have been for her to see me that way.

When we got home, we ate a fabulous meal she had learned at her most recent raw food seminar. We shared a wonderful raw bruschetta appetizer, a fabulous cashew cream mushroom soup, a big green salad, and a raw brownie for dessert. It felt good to fill up on food made with so much love.

Though we had a rough start, the weekend improved. I continued my healing regimen while Robyn worked. I surprised her with some roses and hoped to connect physically, despite the erectile dysfunction—one of the lingering concerns and reasons to continue at OHI. If the program had helped me regain feeling in my lower limbs, neck and hands, I had hoped the progression would continue throughout the rest of my body.

By the time Sunday night arrived, the decision to return to OHI was obvious. Before I stepped inside the train terminal, Robyn and I shared a teary goodbye. I wanted to assure her that I had made the right choice, for both of us.

"I'll look for ways to put on weight," I promised, "and I'll get a meeting with Pam as soon as I can to see about getting more food."

"You better," she said, only half-joking, and the look in her eye suggested that if I didn't, she would find an artful way to get me to eat more. Robyn always had a plan.

23
GOING DEEPER

I woke Monday morning at OHI and took stock of my condition. Sensation had returned to my arms and legs; my mind was sharper, my balance was better, and I felt a spry limberness in my muscles that I hadn't noticed in more than two years. While I welcomed the changes, my recent trip home made me painfully aware that not all the changes were positive. I was too thin and had to keep myself from wasting away.

I had to eat more calories, but they needed to be the right ones. If raw food and detoxing were the answer to keeping MS inactive, I would have to find a way to consume more food while I was in San Diego. I never wanted to see the terror in Robyn's eyes like the day she saw me in the train station—or when I dropped her on our wedding night.

Asking for more wasn't easy. I didn't want to seem like I was asking for any special favors. I wanted to participate equally with the other missionaries and was determined to adhere to the program's digestion guidelines, related to the lifestyle of the ancient Essene people but rooted in a modern theory of optimal health called "Natural Hygiene." Dating back to the 1830s, this diet emphasized that certain foods have to be combined in a particular way in order for optimal digestion and elimination to take place. OHI had adapted and evolved these dietary and digestive guidelines during their thirty years of operation. It meant I would wait an hour to eat after I drank wheatgrass, and ten to thirty minutes after I drank water, green juice, or rejuvelac. Once I ate sprouts, tomatoes, or nuts, I would have to wait thirty minutes to two hours before I could drink again. Though this might have felt regimented at first, the advantages far outweighed the inconveniences: my body would expend minimal effort to metabolize food and could devote as much energy as possible to healing. But the fact remained—no matter how well I followed the digestion guidelines, I would need more calories.

Surprisingly, I was more nervous to discuss all this with Pam than I had been about asking my boss to roll me off the project in Texas. Other than asking Robyn to marry me and my request to leave Texas, I wasn't used to asking for what I wanted or needed. Before OHI, I had worked so hard to create the illusion of perfection in my life—to make it seem like all was good, even as I lost feeling and spiraled toward paralysis. Now, I couldn't afford to live out of alignment with my truth. I was a rail and I needed help. I reluctantly scheduled a meeting with Pam.

After we caught up and I told her the reason for our meeting, Pam moved to the edge of her chair, and in a calm, deliberate voice, said she would send a memo to the kitchen with her approval for me to have additional food at each meal. She emphasized that guest needs were her top priority, and that if there was anything else she could do to enhance my healing, I should just ask. Again, it hit me how easy it had been to get more food—or anything I needed in life. Just like Texas. All I had to do was ask.

As I walked home after the meeting, I realized that extra food might not be all I needed to continue to heal. I had just finished Norman Walker's book on the benefits of green juice and realized the recipe he had developed specifically for people with MS might be the answer to my increased nutritional needs. I had juiced exclusively on Monday through Thursday, but OHI's juice recipe was primarily developed for guests with a wide range of nutritional needs. It wasn't prepared specifically to help me, so while I was augmenting my diet, I decided to add Dr. Walker's vegetable juice recipe.

I wasn't just taking the juice the institute was handing out, I was creating my own. I would need to grocery shop once a week and buy a special juicer, now that I needed to juice five pounds of cucumber, celery, spinach, dandelion, ginger, and burdock root a few times each week—all to get the extra calories I needed to rebuild my body.

Later that week, I had another MS "meeting." The discussions had grown monotonous, and I had taken the previous week off to see if the break provided renewed vigor, or to see if I should stop the conversations altogether. I knew I would be exposed to many ways of healing at OHI and realized some would be more useful than others. The Parts Model might have run its course, but I gave it one last try.

I focused the discussion on one simple question. What did I need to do to continue healing? I asked the question four times. After each inquiry, I sat silently, waiting to hear the answer. I received four answers: I only needed to do this exercise once a week; I needed to respect MS; I needed to bring more joy into my life; and I needed to tap into a passion. I didn't try to rationalize or judge any of the insights but knew I'd need to consider them, and to try and understand how they might relate to my healing.

After the session, I wrote in my journal to reflect, getting clear that I was to continue to meet with the MS once a week for the foreseeable future. I also considered the 'respect the MS' insight, and its meaning was just as clear. I needed to respect myself and not judge my intuitive thoughts.

When I considered passion and joy, their meaning wasn't as clear, and required more reflection. I knew I needed to live my life in alignment with activities that brought excitement and made me happy. I realized I hadn't had much passion (other than being with Robyn) or joy in my life. Work used to be a source of both, but it had become a source of obligation and duty as my health declined. Bike rides and runs had been another source of joy and passion, but as my health worsened, I wasn't able to exercise. The starkest realization was that my relationship with Robyn and my mission to heal were my only current sources of joy and passion, which led me to a dark conclusion: I would have to change my profession if I wanted to live a great life. The thought made me anxious. I had no idea how to do it. The idea was too big; I found solace in the fact that I had two more months to immerse myself in my healing cocoon before I would have to deal.

Over the next few weeks, I searched for more answers by reading a lot. My mother had given me a copy of *Inner Peace* by Parmahansa Yogananda, in my Christmas stocking four years earlier. She thought it might help me find a spiritual influence as I dealt with MS. At the time, I tossed the gift onto my bookshelf—I hadn't been ready to receive the wisdom contained within its pages until I got to OHI. I had packed it before I left home to begin my missionary stay because I knew I would have more time there for spiritual exploration. I decided to read a passage before I went to sleep each night and after I woke each morning to infuse my mind with peace. The book became a trusted spiritual advisor over the remainder of my stay.

Another book I read was *Nature's First Medicine* by Steve Meyerowitz. It provided me with new insights into the three most therapeutic roles of wheatgrass: blood purification, liver detoxification, and colon cleansing. I also learned that fresh wheatgrass was full of life-sustaining vitamins, minerals, and nutrients. According to Charles Schnabel, the father of wheatgrass, fifteen pounds of wheatgrass was equal in nutritional value to 350 pounds of ordinary green vegetables.

Schnabel's work with grass had created a health movement in the 1930's, and dehydrated wheatgrass was apparently found in pharmacies across America as an early multivitamin.

The book also taught me that chlorophyll-rich wheatgrass was a catalyst for the body's ability to heal itself. According to Ann Wigmore, one of the founders of OHI, "[wheat]grass contained all the elements that the body was composed of including revitalizing and rebuilding materials, force producers for energy and eliminators of waste." Clearly, wheatgrass was good for my own body, but I wondered why our culture had moved away from its healing powers.

During my read-athon at OHI, I received an excited phone call from Robyn. She said she had trouble going to sleep the previous night and had wandered up to my office to see if she could find something to read to put her to sleep. She found two books full of underlines and notes in my bookcase. The first was titled *Enzyme Nutrition* by Richard Howell, and the second was *The Colon Health Handbook* by Robert Gray—the two books I picked up in the health food store soon after I was diagnosed, I reminded her.

"That's crazy, it seems like you knew about this path all along," she said.

I had forgotten about those books, but they described our current lifestyle perfectly. It struck me that none of this might have been a coincidence. It was clear that the way our life had unfolded since we had met five years earlier was meant to be.

During lunch one afternoon that week, I sat on the front lawn eating tomatoes, cucumber, celery, and sprouts with Joanne, my missionary friend. I felt the sun's warm, healing rays and excitedly shared my progress. She was impressed with my improvement and asked how I felt about my healing.

"I'm pleased and grateful," I said, "but I need to go deeper."

That's when she told me about a doctor she planned to see later that afternoon— Dr. Edgar Willis, who helped people improve their health by clearing energy blockages using bio cranial therapy to properly align the body.

When I heard he was a chiropractor, I immediately became skeptical. Since I was a kid, I didn't trust chiropractors. I had heard that their bone-cracking techniques had the potential to do permanent damage, so I had never been to one. Before my time at OHI, I never would have gone to see him because I only trusted traditional western medicine. At the institute, I had come to realize that the western medical community was one of many paths to health. Since I was on a healing journey and was open to trying anything that might lead to improved health, I suspended my skepticism and made an appointment. What could it hurt, as long as I didn't let him do any cracking?

During my initial visit, Dr. Willis confirmed what I had heard from Joanne and provided me with greater insight into the healing art. The treatment would release blocked energy in the neck where the spine and neck met and allow cerebral spinal fluid to flow. Apparently, traditional chiropractic only dealt with misalignments in the spine, which constituted only about twenty percent of the central nervous system (CNS). Bio cranial, however, helped clear blockages throughout the *entire* CNS.

I liked what I heard, but had one critical question.

"Do you do any cracking?"

"I don't. I do a stretch of the neck and shoulder to do the adjustment."

He lined up my feet and immediately noticed my left and right legs were out of alignment. "Did you know your left leg is a half inch shorter than your right?"

I was shocked. I had never lined my legs up like that before, and never noticed they rested at different lengths when I lay on my back.

"I didn't. What does that mean?" I asked.

He continued the exam with a muscle test to find other areas where I might have blockages in energy flow. I had never done a muscle test before and asked how it worked. I didn't see any sophisticated electronic monitoring equipment in his office. Apparently there was no need. Muscle testing was a form of muscle-assisted biofeedback that tests body imbalances. It works by testing a person's reaction to various stimuli: a strong response means a healthy reaction, a weak one denotes opportunity for improvement.

"That's it?" I said, not withholding my disbelief.

"Yes, you will be able to see the quality of response for yourself."

Dr. Willis asked me to stand, and proceeded with the tests. He identified a number of places on my upper and lower spine where my strength was diminished and energy was blocked. Then he did a subtle but firm stretch of my trapezius muscles that connected my head and neck. The treatment was brief and before I knew it, he was done.

After he finished, he lined up my legs to see if the stretch made a difference. I could see that my right and left legs were the same length. I was amazed but remained guarded while the doctor continued the exam.

Then he muscle tested me again. I could see the strength in my arm improve. It seemed like a switch had been flicked and the energy was flowing. If I hadn't just experienced the almost instantaneous increase in strength for myself, and seen the evening out of my legs, I wouldn't have thought the stretch made any difference. I was still skeptical about what happened. However, as I walked out of his office, my steps felt more solid and I knew our short time together had made me stronger.

The alternative treatments I had begun to explore also stretched my mind. I began to spend a lot more time meditating after hearing Kimberly mention that Thomas Edison and Albert Einstein used meditation to help them solve problems. The ritual involved diving into a deep soothing meditation for about 30 minutes, and setting the intention to remember my first thought upon 'waking.' On one occasion, I remember coming out of a meditation fixated on my priorities. They needed some serious realignment, too.

Over the previous four years, my priorities had been work, Robyn, and athletics; however, healing was to be my highest priority now, followed by Robyn, and then work.

This re-prioritization made a lot of sense based on the insight I received during my recent MS coaching session, but I wasn't sure whether the new order would jive when I returned home, and later when I returned to work, if I returned at all—a scenario too harrowing for me at the time so I refused to think it. But this re-ordering of priorities was probably the most significant insight to date through my meditation practice. Even more surprising, I didn't judge it or indulge my rational mind by giving it any more thought. I simply wrote the new prioritization in my journal and went to bed. Health came first.

♦

That weekend, I remained at OHI, one of the few weekends that I didn't go home or that Robyn didn't come down to see me. I worked in the garden on Saturday morning to complete my eighteen hours of service for the week. On Sunday, I did laundry, bought vegetables to juice for the following week, did a colonic, and meditated.

I started the next week in a good place. Early one morning, while I did my balance and strength exercises, I had a breakthrough on my Reebok TIS board. A TIS board is an 18" by 30" platform coated with rubber grooves to grip the soles of my shoes that swivels on a ball joint. The board's purpose was to improve my strength and balance.

I would start the exercise with my feet in the middle of the board, about six inches apart, with a solid sense of balance. I would then move my right leg to the board's right outer edge and shift my weight onto that leg. With my feet shoulders-width apart, I moved my right foot back to the center of the board and placed it right next to my left so my feet touched. I would then do the same thing to the left side.

The hard part of the exercise was steadying myself as I shifted my weight. Just lifting my leg to the board's edge could throw me off balance and cause me to fall, but I felt strong and steady enough to cross my right foot in front of my left and extend it all the way to the board's left outer edge. I crossed my legs and shifted my weight through my hips rather than stop in the middle to steady myself. It was a major accomplishment.

Before I arrived at OHI, I had the strength, agility, and balance of an elderly man. When I had started the exercise a few weeks earlier, it was all I could do to maintain my balance and keep from falling off the board as I shuffled my feet and shifted my weight. It hadn't hit me until that morning that I had regained the ability to shift my weight without the need to stop and steady myself *after each step*. I stood in the early afternoon sun and felt a warmth radiate through my whole body. I was getting better.

◆

The healing continued during a hot-rock massage later that same week. My therapist, Catherine, placed fifty half-dollar-sized, smooth lava rocks that had been heated in a Crock-Pot, on my back to loosen my muscles. At one point, she massaged my feet, and I felt a tickle. I couldn't remember the last time I had that sensation. As I lay on the table, I understood how well my body responded to the diet and detox program, the mind-body-spirit unification, the daily yoga and exercise, as well as the emotional exploration. I had listened to my MS and augmented the program with healing insights I had stumbled upon along the way, such as head shakes, balance- and strength-building exercises, placing my hands on heated surfaces, and juicing. My weight loss had stopped, and I had even gained a few pounds. By the end of the hour-long massage, my muscles pulsed with energy. All of this had filled me with optimism that I was on my way to renewed health. I couldn't wait to tell Robyn about my latest healing developments.

I immediately called, and when she answered, I rushed to tell her about my hot rock massage, but she wasn't interested; she needed to talk. It took me a few moments to tune into her apparent crisis, and I felt like a fool. "How was your day?" I finally asked.

"It sucked."

"What happened?"

"It started first thing. I was late for work, so I didn't have anything to eat before I left the house. From the minute I walked into the salon, I had back-to-back clients until after two."

"Did you eat?"

"I finally got some food at two-thirty, but I had passed the hunger point and only ate half my food."

"That stinks."

"Well, that just set me off. I came home tonight to get some dinner, but there wasn't anything to eat. I'm so frustrated; frustrated that I had to come home to an empty house, frustrated that I couldn't find anything to eat, frustrated that we've turned our lives upside down."

Her frustration hadn't yet led to an ultimatum, but our lives had changed drastically. We had cleaned the cupboards of the staples of our SAD (standard American diet) like canned soups, pasta, and rice and had replaced them with only minimal raw food essentials. We had just bought a dehydrator, and Robyn had begun to sprout grain seeds in an attempt to fill her diet. Our raw lifestyle was still very much a work-in-progress at home and took an enormous amount of time to follow. I was fortunate to have my food prepared for me by the OHI staff and missionaries and knew Robyn wasn't so lucky. She was on her own, so when she went to get a bite to eat, she was constantly reminded of our decision.

As I listened, it became painfully obvious that the change in our lifestyle, while beneficial to my health, was hard on Robyn, and I felt bad for what I was putting her through. I was no longer worried about my ability to heal, but if our marriage would survive my choice to do so.

24

EVEN DEEPER

The next day, I picked strawberries on a warm, sunny late-June morning while sparrows chirped overhead. As I placed the plump, ripe fruit into my basket, I noticed the responsiveness in my fingertips. Not only did I have improved dexterity, I could feel the seeds and fuzz. It had been a long time since my fingers felt those sensations. This was very different from the night Robyn carried me to the bathroom or the morning she had to button my shirt for work. How could I feel so good and so bad simultaneously?

I weeded and wondered how much longer I could or should stay at OHI given its strain on Robyn. I thought I was clear on my reworked priorities: healing, Robyn, and work. They sounded great on paper, but implementing them would be an entirely new challenge. Robyn had been vital to my recovery. She was still trying to live 100% raw for me. She was my biggest cheerleader, her counsel grounded me, her food rebuilt me, and her love made me complete. I would've been a hopeless, helpless mess without her, and I worried that my prolonged stay at OHI might eventually break us down.

I considered if I should end my time eight weeks early to return to her, but since the program had improved my health and given me hope, the idea of leaving early was the last thing I wanted. I wanted that concrete feeling of recovery. I had to believe this was not an either-or situation. I wanted to achieve both—healing and a healthy marriage.

I returned to my apartment and immediately called Robyn. I asked her if she still felt the frustration from the previous night. She said she had a good day. Relieved, I told her I needed to find some way to continue healing, but it couldn't be at the expense of our relationship. She agreed, and we decided to see each other more often. We decided to spend each weekend together until I completed my stay.

I hung up and the pit in my stomach was gone.

The next day, I pulled weeds in the garden and thought about the book I was reading, *The Healing Sun, Sunlight and Health in the 21st Century*, by Richard Hobday. Its pages were dense and debunked numerous beliefs that had filled my mind since I was a kid. The biggest was the myth that the sun was a source of dread—a belief imprinted on me as a six-year-old kid in Vermont.

I sat in the front seat of our big blue Buick station wagon. I had won the prized position after a hard-fought battle with Pete. He was two years older and bigger, so I didn't win those battles often. We were stopped at a traffic light, and I gazed up at the sun for a few seconds, then I turned back to Pete and triumphantly announced, "I just stared at the sun."

"That's dangerous," he barked from the backseat. "You shouldn't do that. You could go blind."

I didn't have any reason to think differently until that week at OHI. *The Healing Sun* was full of knowledge. It reminded me that the sun was the source of all life but also contained shocking concepts that altered my view of it. The most radical was that the sun could be used as medicine to heal and prevent numerous diseases, multiple sclerosis included. There was one important caveat; sun exposure had to be used correctly. Using the sun as medicine was a gradual process that needed to be introduced slowly and at the right times of the day so that it didn't do damage.

As much as I wanted to believe the radical claims exposed, I needed more proof. The author hadn't included any scientific studies to back up his conclusions. He gave only anecdotal evidence—stories of babies healed of jaundice and children cured of tuberculosis almost a hundred years earlier. The sun's ability to heal jaundice was now commonly accepted by Western Medicine, and I accepted the less-than-perfect theory that the sun could help me heal, too.

That same week, I happened upon an Indian man named "HRN" featured in a flyer promoting a seminar on solar healing he was teaching in San Diego. The talk was scheduled for the coming weekend. I planned to attend the wedding of one of Robyn's friends that weekend, so unfortunately I would miss it, but I wondered if maybe "HRN" would help me understand the healing power of the sun.

That weekend, I returned to Santa Monica to attend the wedding with Robyn. My first night back, I hopped online to look into solar healing. I found that "HRN" stood for Hira Ratan Manek, a retired engineer from India who had rediscovered that the body uses the pineal gland to harness the sun's power. On his official website, HRN explained how to use the sun to heal. I was surprised by its simplicity. He said that the process should begin by staring for only ten seconds per day, then increasing exposure by ten-second increments daily. He stressed that a person must only look at the sun up until an hour after it rose or starting an hour before it set, when UV radiation was zero. Levels above zero caused harm to the eyes and could lead to blindness. My brother had been right.

According to HRN, once a person reached thirty minutes of continuous gazing, his outer body would be healed of disease. He listed two dozen illnesses that would respond favorably—one was multiple sclerosis. HRN also made a more radical claim. He said after a person reached forty-five minutes of consecutive gazing that their appetite would diminish and that their body could run on sunlight and water alone.

HRN reported that he had completed fasts up to 411 days long by living only on water and the sun. A team of medical experts and scientists from around the world observed his second fast and corroborated his radical findings.

I had heard about the pineal gland while at OHI and knew it was commonly referred to as the third eye—a center of spiritual enlightenment and intuition, but I was still skeptical. The more I looked into HRN's approach, the more my rational mind objected. Staring at the sun to heal my body sounded outlandish.

I thought the best place for this information was the trash can. It was late and I was tired. I shut down the computer and went to sleep. I hoped my subconscious would make sense of what I read, but I was still baffled the next morning.

By the time we arrived at the rehearsal dinner in Long Beach, I had forgotten what I had read the night before. Robyn spent Saturday morning with the bridal party, so I had the time to myself. I meditated, wrote in my journal, and read. After two hours alone in my room, I needed fresh air, and I decided to see how far my body would carry me and took a walk around the harbor.

Before my time at OHI, I had been reluctant to walk distances longer than a quarter mile for fear that my body would give out. But that morning, I walked about two miles. Later that night, I danced with Robyn for the first time since our wedding. Though my steps were stilted, it felt good to feel the rhythm of the music and move as a couple again.

As Robyn drove me to the train station at the end of our weekend together, it occurred to me to bring up the sun gazing to see what she thought. I knew it was a radical idea and had the possibility to sever the connection we had just reestablished, but after all I had done to rebuild my body at OHI, I wanted to give sun gazing a shot and wanted to make sure she knew about it.

"I think I've found a new healing technique that might take my healing deeper."

"What's that?" she asked.

"Sun gazing."

Robyn turned to me, perplexed. "I've never heard of that."

"It involves staring at the sun when there is no UV radiation to damage the eyes."

"That doesn't sound safe. What do you have to do?"

"Not much. This guy from India stumbled across the technique, and it's just beginning to gain acceptance."

"By who? Crazy, kooky monkeys? You're in a good place with your healing. Are you sure you want to add something that might take you in an unknown direction? Why are you always looking for the next thing? I think you need to focus on what you're already doing and master that."

I wanted to tell her about its powerful potential, but I bit my tongue to end the discord. We said our good-byes, and I boarded the train back to San Diego. My body was tired, but a good tired. I stared out the window in a dream-like daze for most of the ride, re-living the weekend, the walk around the harbor, the reception, and dancing with Robyn. As the stations passed, I realized how much I wanted to be able to dance into old age and live happily and independently with my wife. I wondered if I was doing enough to make that happen.

Would the sun round out my recovery? Other than HRN's claims, I had found no proof that sunlight could do anything to improve MS. I knew experientially the sun could have a positive effect on my condition when I put my hands on the sidewalk and the warmth of the sun seemed to help awaken feeling in my hands, but that wasn't very scientific. I had already pursued a number of questionable healing techniques, and they all had one thing in common: each was based on a simple life truth. The body is programmed to return to its natural state of optimal health if you surround it with a supportive environment and provide the right things: food, water, air, and thoughts.

Why couldn't the sun be an ally, too? All life on earth was powered by the sun, either directly through photosynthesis, or indirectly through the web of life. I wondered if humans were always meant to receive a portion of their energy directly from the sun, and if HRN had simply rediscovered the mechanism that had remained dormant in humans for ages. I concluded that I had nothing to lose, and maybe a lot to gain, from sun gazing.

♦

After dinner the first night back at OHI, I went down to the garden at sunset to begin my sun gazing practice. I remembered the time the sun had gone down the previous night, and I found myself among the plants a few minutes before then. It was very peaceful that time of day as birds sang and vegetables grew. I found a good spot in the front row next to some tomato plants. I was out of the view of guests, behind a hedge that separated the garden from the parking lot. I usually didn't care if others witnessed my peculiar healing behavior, but that day I was self-conscious because of Robyn's opinions.

Sun gazing crossed the line of what *I* considered socially acceptable and wasn't sure how long I'd continue the practice. HRN's website said that if I made it to thirty minutes of continuous gazing, my body would be healed. This meant that I'd have to sun gaze every day for 180 days consecutively, increasing the duration ten seconds per day. That was half a year, if I gazed every day per week. I imagined I'd have no problem doing that during the eight weeks I had left as a missionary, but I wasn't sure if I could maintain the schedule once I returned home. Even so, I didn't let that stop me.

I lifted my head and stared at the sun. As I looked, I counted to ten by one-thousands. In the time it took my eyes to adjust to the light, I was done. When I finished, I closed my eyes for a few seconds and allowed them to adjust. The whole experience happened quickly. If anyone had seen me, I imagined it looked like I had taken a brief look toward the horizon to catch a glimpse of the sunset. Nothing uncommon happened. I wasn't suddenly struck by lightning, nor did I have an incredible flash of awareness.

That night I called Robyn to tell her I had sun gazed, even though I knew she wasn't comfortable with the idea. I wanted to tell her the truth but hoped I would get voice mail. I had no such luck. She answered on the second ring.

I tried to offer her more than my first pitch before the train ride. I reiterated in depth that sun gazing held the promise to heal a number of diseases, multiple sclerosis included. I hoped to soften her before I shared the most controversial benefit: people who sun gazed could refrain from eating for periods of up to a year by subsisting on water and sunlight alone. The line went silent.

"I still don't think it's a good idea," Robyn said. I'm sure what she wanted to say was, Are *you fucking kidding me?! After all we've been through and the weight loss?! Sun?*

"I've done research into how to gaze so I won't do damage. There's a watch I can get that measures UV radiation that I'm going to buy this week."

"Jon, no. I don't think you understand how much I worry. I'm not okay with it. I'm scared of anything that might lead to more weight loss or worse, damage your eyes, but do what you have to do."

Matt had told me the same thing when I walked away from our start-up venture.

Four years later, Robyn would tell me she thought the idea of staring at the sun sounded insane, but she didn't put her foot down because she didn't want to impede my healing. Other than her initial feeling about OHI before our visit, this was the only time that Robyn and

I really differed in our view of healing. I didn't see any downside. HRN's protocol seemed safe. I liked how easy it was to do and was determined to continue.

Later that week, I had a bio cranial appointment with Dr. Willis. He invited me into the treatment room and asked how things were going.

"Great." I answered with some hesitation in my voice, and then told him about using sun gazing to heal. Coincidentally, he had just heard HRN speak at the seminar.

I was so excited to hear Dr. Willis knew about it and didn't think it was some crazy, whacked-out practice and had even tried it himself. He told me about the watch he had ordered to measure UV radiation and I was even more excited to get one, too.

The instances of synchronicity continued that week when a guest named Grace Maverick approached me as I finished dinner one night and introduced herself. I assumed that, based on her name alone, she might have something insightful to share. She told me she had overheard me talk about the power of the program with a guest during lunch that afternoon and apparently had decided to extend her stay by a day to speak to me. She went on to tell me about the power of belief and asked if I was open to her insights.

"Of course," I replied. It seemed strange that she would extend her stay just to speak with me before we'd even met, but I was open to hearing anything she might know about healing. She told me about a book she thought I'd like called *The Biology of Belief,* that theorized the environment, rather than genetics, determines our health.

Clearly my prior environments at work and at school were not positive for my health. Immersed in them, I had chosen to push myself beyond my limits. I had no boundaries, and I didn't know it was my responsibility to define them and make the appropriate and necessary changes so that my environment would support me, not cause my collapse. Before the diagnosis, I thought that pushing my limits was a part of living a great life. I had accomplished a lot and was living a great life on paper (successful, according to some), but I wasn't emotionally in touch with what I really needed. Clearly, something was amiss in my world and had been for a very long time.

But there was hope. Grace emphasized that I wasn't destined for a life of disease. I had the power to experience an alternative future if I believed it was possible, but I had the responsibility to co-create the right environment.

As I sat and talked with Grace, I understood that while many people are hit by "shit storms," how you walked through yours determined your fate. I was ready to do whatever it took to recreate the supportive conditions at OHI in order to heal at home.

25

CHANGING MY ENVIRONMENT
INSIDE AND OUT

In the beginning of July, I took the Pacific Surfliner train home to celebrate our first wedding anniversary. In less than a year, Robyn and I had been married, bought a house, made major renovations, watched my health deteriorate, and found a way for me to heal—there was a lot to celebrate.

We arrived home from the station to enjoy the scrumptious four-course raw food meal that Robyn had prepared. Mushroom soup, bruschetta, walnut loaf, salad, and a dessert of chocolate mouse. Robyn had gotten into the swing of preparing raw food. Shortly after we sat to eat, we heard a *crack-crack* and then a loud boom. Startled, we followed the noise upstairs and popped out on the roof deck to see the sky filled with fireworks for Santa Monica's Fourth of July celebration.

The sky filled with light was an unexpected gift. Robyn stood in front of me and I held her tight. I couldn't think of a better way to celebrate our anniversary. After the finale, we went back down to finish dinner and exchange gifts. I gave Robyn a framed photo from our wedding and a sexy negligee, and she gave me a framed picture from our honeymoon and negligee for her to wear. We both laughed because we hadn't shared what we planned to give each other.

The photo I'd given Robyn showed us standing alone at our reception in the grand ballroom entry. The photo captured Robyn's steady strength amidst chaos, which had served us well through the challenges of our first year of marriage.

The photo Robyn gave me showed us alone in our bathing suits on the beach, celebrating our honeymoon on the private island of Petit St. Vincent in the Caribbean, a vision of the prosperous and healthy life Robyn hoped we'd share. But since then, I had lost my health, and as much as I wanted to give her the man in the photo—a guy with unbridled enthusiasm for our future—I wasn't ready. I needed to return to OHI and continue to heal, no matter how hard it would be to leave her again.

I returned to San Diego and at the end of another week of healing, I found myself seated in front of a room full of guests. It was Friday morning and testimony time at the institute. This was the only instance when the director approved of people speaking about their conditions. Guests would talk about how much weight they'd lost, how they had reduced their blood pressure, or how they'd lowered their PSA levels and were out of the danger zone with prostate cancer. I shared my testimony: after nearly three months of experiencing continuous small changes in my body, I had seen significant recovery. I walked with full strides now, feeling had returned to my hands and feet, the tingling had almost completely subsided, and my speech was fluid. The program had worked.

That weekend, I was so excited to take time away from OHI and connect with Robyn. I missed her during the week and couldn't wait to see her. She planned to drive us to Jacumba, a small desert town on the Mexican border, world-renowned for the healing power of its desert hot springs. I had heard about the place from a guest at the institute and reserved a room at the only motel in town that piped the spring water right into a tub in our suite. I couldn't wait to see her and just *be* with her.

She arrived at OHI to pick me up, and we headed east on I-8 into the desert. Twenty miles into our trip, strip malls and suburban track homes gave way to cacti and yucca plants. The late afternoon sun bathed the landscape in a deep orange glow. I was struck by the desert beauty and solitude. Robyn turned to me as we drove.

"Tell me about your week. What did you learn?"

I stared out at the passing cacti. I wanted to tell her that I had sun gazed each day and that my brief sessions staring at the sun had been very relaxing and centering, like abbreviated meditation sessions that offered the same benefits as a full twenty minutes. Because I hadn't figured out how to talk about sun gazing so that she'd be okay with it, I didn't mention it and chose something safe instead.

"I read a great passage from *Inner Peace*."

"Tell me."

I told her how Yogananda believed people should marry only after they learned how to handle their emotions. I realized how emotionally illiterate I had been before OHI when it came to expressing negative feelings of anger, fear, and loneliness. I obviously didn't have the tools to process those feelings at the time and buried them instead. Robyn didn't take well to my "latest insight."

"You know how ironic that is, right?"

I hadn't intended my comment to be any reflection on our marriage or imply that we had somehow made a mistake. "I just mean to say that I'm learning how much I need to work on expressing my emotions," I said, hoping she would see my earnestness. I didn't want to argue; I wanted to enjoy our short time together.

"Okay. I get it. What's the significance?" she asked.

"I'm not really sure. It probably has something to do with not wanting to discuss negative or bad things."

"I can understand wanting to avoid the negative, but you know sometimes those feelings need to be expressed so you can let them out."

"Yeah, I'm starting to get what that means."

I had become so engrossed in our discussion that I didn't realize the hour-and-a-half trip was over until we'd exited the highway, drove through Jacumba, and stopped at our motel. Inside our room, I walked toward the back door that led to the deck and passed a mirror, noticing how tan and healthy I looked. The weight loss had stopped and I had gained about five pounds since the night Robyn greeted my emaciated body at the train station, and I looked very different than the pale, bloated body I had back in April.

I stepped onto the patio, excited to soak up the volcanic waters in the hot tub, already feeling the expansiveness of the outdoors. I climbed a chair to look over the back wall and survey the sparse desert landscape, glimpsing the border fence that ran up a ridge and separated the U.S. from Mexico. I saw the setting sun cast long shadows that revealed a landscape wrinkled like an accordion; the natural beauty was striking, and I felt close to the land. A wave of euphoria hit me like it did when I picked strawberries.

Later that night, Robyn and I walked to dinner holding hands.

"This place is cool," Robyn said.

I squeezed her hand. "It feels so right."

Before we walked into the hotel bar to get salads to augment the raw foods Robyn had brought in the cooler, we stopped at the front desk to find the location of the onsite massage therapist. We also bumped into the owner, who gave us a brief history of the place and told us there had been a group of monks at the motel the previous week. He said the hot springs were the best in the country and drew people to tiny Jacumba from around the world. He expressed his belief that Jacumba had a strong divine connection.

Before my time at OHI, I was not attuned to spiritual intuition; divine insights would have passed through me like water, and I would have dismissed Jacumba as a crazy hippy town. With our old worldview in command, we probably would have canceled our reservation and driven back to San Diego. Clearly, we had changed.

After two incredible days together, we returned to San Diego rejuvenated and connected to our essence; I was finally out of my head and very in tune with how I felt. We were both present and focused on each other in a place that supported us, and I wondered if it was possible to live such an ideal existence outside these healing cocoons.

The morning after my trip to Jacumba, I woke anxious; I usually started most days calmly writing in my journal, but that morning was different. I sat at my desk and feverishly wrote; my hand struggled to keep up with my mind. A dam had broken. Since becoming a missionary, I had understood the importance of my emotions. That morning my mind wanted to explore the connection between the onset of MS and my emotions, to see if there was a link. I looked back over the eight years since the diagnosis and tried to identify my emotional state during the worst MS attacks. What I found stunned me. The optic neuritis and the basketball court episode that lead to the diagnosis were both associated with considerable emotional upset. It finally made sense.

During the optic neuritis attack, my first semester at MIT, I felt immense pressure to succeed and was driven by an extreme fear of failure. I felt the need to prove I belonged and questioned whether I measured up to the standards set by such a prestigious school. I slept very little for two straight weeks, as I drove myself to make the most of every hour. I didn't allow my body to fully rejuvenate at the end of each day.

During the second episode, I had experienced two emotional traumas. The first was the result of my personal demons—the belief that I had to prove myself with my graduate thesis—the same stress that I felt during the optic neuritis episode a year earlier. The second trauma was the breakup of a serious year-and-a-half-long relationship with a woman, which I had handled immaturely. Rather than work through my feelings of doubt about our relationship, I ignored them and just broke up with her. I shut the door and never looked back. Since we ended things on that cold snowy day in February of 1997, we've never talked. I'm still sorry about the way I handled this and would do things differently today—but this illustrated once again how the emotions I had trapped inside me contributed to the MS attacks.

About this time, I finished reading *The Biology of Belief*. The book provided scientific evidence of the impact that beliefs had on the body and confirmed what I had grown to know about environmental factors also affecting my health. A key component to a life without MS symptoms was to free myself from emotional and physical stress. I assumed that meant I would need to become good at dealing with unrest as it surfaced. I didn't see how I could completely avoid it and hoped the tools I had learned at OHI would allow me to express my feelings more freely. How I handled my emotions going forward—either experiencing them as a storm or in a calmer, serene way would impact my ability to maintain my well-being.

The 'miracle' to my recovery wasn't any one thing I had done or would do. The key to renewed health was creating harmony in the world around me. But with only a month left at OHI, I was scared I couldn't create the environment I needed for continued good health and healing at home. I thought about the framed anniversary photo of Robyn and me on the Caribbean beach. I desperately wanted to be the "real" guy in the image, and even better, a healthy man in touch with his emotions, not the diseased man with wavering steps, a clouded mind, and waning confidence. Though, I had found my way back to health, I wondered how I would maintain it.

26

TAKING THE BIGGEST RISK

The thought of navigating life without the constant help of OHI scared the hell out of me; I wasn't sure I could do it. Though I knew intuitively that my condition had improved, I needed conventional medicine to confirm that OHI had worked. Since the diagnosis, I appreciated allopathic, or 'western' medicine, for its ability to diagnose illness and disease, even though I wasn't sure it helped to unlock the body's inherent ability to heal.

Three weeks before the end of my OHI stay, I returned home for the weekend and stayed through Monday to get a physical. I looked forward to my yearly appointment with my general practitioner, Dr. Prudente. He was the doctor who had put me on the Lipitor I had stopped taking before I left for OHI. I was anxious to hear what he had to say. The nurse came in and took my vitals. I weighed 140 pounds, which didn't surprise me. My pulse was seventy and blood pressure was 118 over 66. I couldn't remember ever having had such low readings. I hoped the results of my blood work would further substantiate OHI's impact on my health; the corporate guy in me still liked numbers.

"Hey Ernie," I said as the doctor walked in.

"Wow, you're tan. I see you're spending a lot of time outdoors; you're wearing sunscreen, right?"

He asked what I'd done to get such a great tan. I took a minute to bring him up to speed. Ernie was progressive and knew about alternative healing modalities and was impressed by my claims of improved strength and balance while at OHI, but I could see he maintained a healthy skepticism. He checked my skin for unwanted growths or discolorations that might indicate skin cancer. He listened to my heart and lungs, looked at my tonsils, and checked me for testicular cancer. Then he put me through the exact same battery of neurological tests that Dr. Woo would do. I looked forward to this part of the exam. I assumed it would show my improvement.

He finished the tests and we briefly chatted. He commented specifically on my arm and leg strength, as well as my ability to walk on my heels and toes. The heel/toe exercise was the best indication of my improvement because I didn't have the strength or dexterity to walk on them during a neurological exam seven months earlier. His reaction fueled my optimism about a continued recovery.

"I feel I've recovered about 75% and want to heal 100%."

Ernie took a more conservative position. "It's okay if you don't recover 100%. You should be pleased with what you've achieved."

It made me angry to hear I should be okay with anything less than a full recovery, but I didn't want to argue, so I shifted my focus back to the physical. My cholesterol was the only thing that remained a question. I had stopped taking Lipitor after learning that the non-animal fat diet, combined with increased physical activity, would naturally lower cholesterol levels. I was curious to see if that was true but would have to wait for the blood test results to know for sure.

I went home and reported the good news to Robyn, but when I shared the doctor's comment, she slammed her glass on the kitchen counter.

"That's bullshit. He needs to be more encouraging!"

How could I have thought she'd be okay with anything less than a full recovery?

That night I returned to OHI, and the next morning I jumped out of bed to write in my journal and release my frustration. I was angry that the doctor had even introduced the idea of anything less than a full recovery; however, he motivated me to step up my game. I would follow the program to the letter over my final three weeks. This included greater diligence with daily enemas, the program requirement I sometimes skipped.

We had made significant changes at home, totally reconfiguring our kitchen to support my continued healing, but I was still scared that once I left OHI, I would stop healing, and worse, that my health would decline. During my remaining meal conversations, many guests said that life 'outside' OHI would be different, and this terrified me. I was concerned that my friends and coworkers wouldn't understand or accept our new lifestyle.

One night after dinner, a woman approached me and asked if I was the person who had been a guest with her back in April. I recognized her and said I was. Her eyes welled with tears. She said that I looked totally different: I stood upright, spoke clearly, and looked strong and vibrant. She said it was a miracle, and her words made me tingle. It was the reflection I needed to leave OHI, not just with a plan, but with courage.

♦

Ironically, pain bolstered my confidence. At 3 a.m. on the Saturday morning two weeks prior to finishing the program, I woke with an excruciating pain in my neck. It felt like someone had gripped my spine and tried to rip it from my body. The pain lasted about an hour until I fell back asleep; it was the most intense pain I'd ever felt.

When I woke the next morning, I stayed in bed trying to make sense of what happened. I was supposed to be leaving the institute for a weekend with Robyn and my family to celebrate my father's seventy-first birthday. All I wanted to do was think about the fun we had planned for the weekend, but I couldn't get past the pain. I was at a loss for why it occurred; I had done everything the program asked the previous week.

My rational mind looked for an answer, and I assumed it was the result of my body holding onto fear—fear of the future, fear of navigating all the unknowns once I left OHI. Before I got up, I did Kimberly's six-step process to move the fear through my body.

I continued to relax in bed, when an alternative reason for the pain hit me. I hadn't had feeling in the back of my neck since I'd arrived at the institute; I'm not sure when I lost feeling because I'd become increasingly numb over the previous year and a half. I realized that another explanation for the pain was that the nerves in the back of my neck were regaining sensation and coming back to life. This was a good sign of my recovery and the best news I could take home to my family.

When I returned to Santa Monica later that day, I saw a letter from Dr. Prudente on the counter. I ripped it open, finding three pages of blood test results. I did a quick scan, realized my scores were all well within normal, and took a deep breath. Upon closer examination, I saw that my cholesterol count was 121, one percentage point above the low end of normal: 120 to 210. I rushed upstairs to find my previous year's score to compare results: 201. I realized my cholesterol had decreased forty percent in eleven months, and the tingling returned. Because I was on Lipitor for a few months before I left for the institute, I knew the result wasn't totally attributable to my vegan diet and increased exercise, though I also knew that both had helped significantly.

Robyn shared my excitement, but it didn't surprise her. She'd watched me grow stronger and more mentally clear over the previous three months.

"That's great news," she said, preoccupied. She stood in the kitchen, struggling to finish the special dessert she was making so I could have something sweet during my dad's birthday celebration. She wanted to make a 'raw' blueberry cheesecake, but she couldn't find a recipe online. It wasn't like she could open a Duncan Hines cake box, mix the ingredients in a bowl, and pour them into a pan.

I put the test scores down. "Do you need help?" I asked, having no idea how I could assist her.

"Nope."

I watched her work, blowing wisps of blonde hair out of her eyes. I was awed by her determination, remembering her initial aversion to raw food. Here she was diving into the alchemy of raw food preparation—trying to create a 'raw' cheesecake, not an easy task from the looks of it. She'd been at this for a while, approaching the challenge like a scientist. She tinkered with everything she could to get the texture and flavor just right.

Tonight, she was on the verge of a breakthrough, and I was witnessing it. She'd finally figured out a way for the 'raw' cake to maintain its shape by using the perfect ingredient: psyllium husk, which allowed the cake to hold its form.

I probably stood over her a bit too long, amazed by her focus.

"What?" she said, looking up with a hint of pride in her eyes.

"You're amazing," I said.

"You haven't tried it yet. That's the real test."

I shook my head and smiled, thinking, *Here is my beautiful wife making me a cake that I can eat.* I had never considered I would one day be able to enjoy a treat like this, given the strict adherence to my diet. It wasn't just the raw cheesecake that filled me with an immense sense of well-being and hope. Robyn was working hard, using her creative gifts, to make my transition from OHI a success.

The next day we drove to Santa Barbara with Robyn's raw invention positioned safely in the backseat and joined my parents at the Spiritland Bistro to celebrate my dad's birthday. My dad had decided on the restaurant because it satisfied our family's broad spectrum of tastes, from meat and potatoes to raw/vegan. I was impressed with how my parents embraced our new lifestyle. It felt good to be able to go out to a restaurant with my wife and parents and order from the menu. Our salads, appetizers, and main courses were amazing, but the featured course was Robyn's dessert.

The wait staff placed a slice of cheesecake in front of each of us. I ogled the inch-and-a-half-thick wedge of blueberry cake with sauce oozing down the side. When we each had a plate, I took a bite and was immediately overcome by delight. Robyn's creation was rich and smooth, just like real cheesecake. Conversation around the table stopped as we each relished her dessert. My mom was the first to speak.

"WOW, it's delicious. So rich and smooth!" she said.

We were all awed by how Robyn was able to make foods with the texture, taste, and look she wanted by using all raw, unprocessed ingredients. Our comments evolved into an energized discussion about the creation of a raw cheesecake company. As we spoke, the manager, chef, and our server came to the table. Robyn had told the staff they could eat the half they didn't serve us.

"Who made the cake?" the chef asked with a very serious look on his face.

"I did," Robyn responded, sheepishly. "What do you think?"

The chef smiled.

"We loved it! And it looked just like a regular piece of cheesecake."

Her experiment with the psyllium husk as the coagulant had worked.

"Yeah, without all of the bad stuff," Robyn said and smiled at me.

"We are onto something big," I wrote in my journal later that night, having no idea that Robyn's experimental raw cheesecake would launch her culinary career and play a key role in our future harmony and prosperity.

◆

After our magical weekend, I returned to OHI and settled into my routine for my final two weeks. All I could think about was the passage I had read and copied into my journal from *Inner Peace* during my train ride back: *Peace is a beautiful quality. We should pattern our life by a triangular guide: calmness and sweetness are two sides; the base is happiness. Whether one acts quickly or slowly, in solitude or in the busy marts of men, his center should be peaceful, poised.*

As I reviewed the words, it hit me. If I could maintain calm, thoughtful intentions, and stay happy as the chaos of the world moved around me, I could stay enveloped in a healing peace. It seemed naive and way too simple to be true, but I knew in my heart that Yogananda's words were an important piece of the puzzle to maintaining my health. I just needed to figure out how to find that peace in the "real" world.

The following weekend, prior to my last week at OHI, I returned home to Robyn and another great raw dinner she had prepared. We shared a spirited conversation as we ate, talking about life after OHI. We discussed having a baby, and Robyn expressed her fear and uncertainty about whether we'd have a healthy baby. She was worried about genetics. She spoke about our chances of passing MS to a baby. I was more concerned with whether I'd be able to provide for a family.

Before we were engaged, we had talked about kids; we both wanted them badly, but during the year since then, talk of babies was taboo. We'd decided against starting a family when my health started deteriorating. It was a sad reality. I could barely care for myself, much less a child, and there was no way I wanted Robyn burdened by being a caretaker *and* mother. But now that I was improving, we could finally address the taboo.

As we talked that night about the creation of a stable, secure environment to bring a child into the world, I became resistant. I was scared. I took my role as provider seriously. I'd have to return to my job but wasn't sure that particular environment would allow me to continue to heal. Mostly, I wasn't sure if I could deliver on what it meant to provide for a family and heal at the same time.

I woke my final morning at OHI, wrote in my journal, and meditated. Then I scurried up the hill for exercise; on my way, I stopped and juiced wheatgrass. It was surreal to go through my last early-morning routine. It felt like yesterday that I had limped across campus with Robyn on the welcome tour.

My body moved differently now. I led the group twice around campus during exercise and navigated the narrow path by the pool without wavering. After my workout, I found a seat in the front of the room for Friday morning circle and my graduation ceremony. I sat patiently as the room filled to capacity—my family among them.

My parents, brother, and Robyn had all traveled to attend my graduation. They'd had to sneak into the ceremony because it was meant for guests only. If questioned, they had planned to ask for forgiveness. I caught Pete's eye and gave him a nod of gratitude. I wouldn't have been there had he not planted the seed back in January. My family had played a critical role in my recovery, and I was honored they made the trip.

For the first half hour of the ceremony, we recognized guests who'd completed their three-week program and then acknowledged the service of missionaries, who had finished their three-month commitment. When the audience clapped to acknowledge our service, I stood and scanned the room. I caught the eye of several guests who I'd connected with and a wave of sorrow hit me; I'd miss our mealtime conversations. The discussions had been such an invaluable source of inspiration and insight. I would need to find new sources of ideas and encouragement at home.

The highlight of the morning came next, when guests volunteered to share their stories. I raised my hand when testimonials began but wasn't called on until last, since it was my final day. When it was finally my turn, I stood and took a seat front and center,

"My name is Jon Chandonnet," I said, "and I just completed three months as a missionary."

I paused and looked around, the room. It was completely silent. I talked about the diagnosis, about how I'd lived six and a half years symptom-free. I spoke about how MS had taken hold of me and how I had gone into a two-year period of terror and decline. I shared how my condition had become so bad that I could barely walk, talk, think, or feel. I described how I'd totally lost hope, before I made the decision to attend OHI.

I spoke unrehearsed and completely from my heart.

I spoke through tears of joy about the recovery that I had experienced, immersed in an environment of love and support. How I'd worked my way back to health, found hope, and in the process, realized something very important—my body could heal itself. As the result of four months at OHI, I came to sense the disease was influenced by what I was putting into my body: food, thoughts, or emotions that had not contributed to my well-being. I explained that eating live, nutrient and enzyme rich food and filling my mind with health affirming thoughts had dramatically improved my condition. If I respected my mind, body, and spirit, embraced my emotions, and lived in harmony with myself and my surroundings, I could heal. I felt stronger, more mentality acute, alive, and balanced than I had in several years except for the afternoon in July 2004 when I said 'I do'.

I watched the mood of the room shift as I shared how my condition had improved.

This was what it meant to live the great life that Dr. Heller had suggested after he gave me the diagnosis eight years earlier. I wished he could have been there to hear the significance of his words. When I finished, I stood and the room erupted in applause; there was hardly a dry eye in the place, including my own. I had found my voice.

27
RETURN HOME

After four months at OHI, I was thinking clearly, walking normal, and no longer feeling numbness or tingling in my hands or legs. I was confident that it was not only possible to keep MS symptoms at bay—it was also possible to reverse the damage, assuming I could construct an equally supportive environment at home.

Despite my optimism, I was anxious. Regressing scared me. I knew it would take time to acclimate to life on the outside, and I assumed my continued recovery would be a work in progress. I just hoped the two weeks before my return to Sapient would be enough time to build a foundation for continued healing.

As I drove up the coast, passing lush fields along the highway, I felt a surge of excitement. I could grow my own wheatgrass! The grass that I had juiced and drank every day at OHI had become an essential part of my renewed health. Growing it myself would keep me in tune with the life cycle I had found in the garden, which I felt was critical to my ongoing recovery. I wanted to continue to drink four ounces per day—the dose recommended by the institute for maintenance. I left OHI with all the knowledge I needed to grow it at home. I wanted to drink the highest quality juice while minimizing its cost.

I soon fantasized about becoming the "wheatgrass guy" of Southern California. My journey back to health, powered by the grass, had opened my eyes to the potentially prosperous idea of creating a chain of juice bars that would allow people to regain and maintain vibrant health. This probably sounds a little delusional, but I was desperate to find a constructive way to occupy my time before going back to work.

Before I got carried away by my grandiose vision, I had to prove that growing wheatgrass would be less expensive than buying it at the local health food store. When I got home, I calculated what it would cost me to buy a year's worth—four ounces per day—at the store. It added up to $1,800 a year—a significant expense. Then I calculated the cost to grow a flat a week at home, which came to $340 a year. I was confident that I could make it work. That night I excitedly shared my plan with Robyn.

"You sure you want to go through all the trouble?" she asked.

"Yeah, it'll be a fun project to pass the time."

"You still plan to go back to work, right?"

"Of course, but it will be good to stay in tune with the earth and maybe save some money. Who knows what it might turn into?"

"Knock yourself out."

On my first morning back, I woke early, eager to continue healing the OHI way. First, I wrote in my journal. I summed up the essence of my turn-around into six core concepts: mind/body/spirit connection, live enzyme-rich raw food, daily exercise, body detoxification, positive affirming beliefs, and emotional expression.

Since I had regained the stride of a healthy thirty-five-year-old male, I learned how to evaluate whether something I added to my routine worked or not. My recovery decisions were guided by a simple premise—if my condition improved or at least held steady after I introduced something new, then I could keep it. If it didn't, I'd toss it out.

My healing hadn't progressed along a straight line from disease to health, so I had learned the importance of patience and not to make rash assumptions about a food or technique before it had time to work. The hard part was to know how long to wait, but I would have to employ this same mentality at home.

There was one big difference between following my regimen as a missionary and creating one at home. At OHI, a few ounces of wheatgrass, a raw meal, a massage, or a yoga class were easy to get. I just had to find the time, schedule the activity, and show up.

At home, I had more demands and would have to find a way to manage my time. My return marked the end of the detoxification phase and the start of the reconstruction phase. It was time to see how I could do both—heal and gain weight while I reconnected with Robyn, strengthened our marriage and regained my professional footing.

With a clear sense of my plan, I headed to the beach to sun gaze. I stepped out of the Jeep, instantly felt a warm ocean breeze, and walked toward the sand. When I arrived at the bike path, I looked back at the eastern horizon to see if the sun had crested the tree line; it hadn't, so I walked out onto the sand in search of a spot to gaze. I found one just before the beach dropped off into the surf.

I removed my shoes and socks, dug my feet into the sand, and felt the cool, moist grains between my toes. I savored the moment because I'd completely lacked feeling below my knees four months earlier. I took a seat and faced the water, listening to the rhythmic pounding of waves. After a few minutes of bliss, I noticed the sun had risen above the trees; it was time.

I stood, rooted my feet, and checked my watch. Since the sun had just risen, its rays wouldn't reach harmful levels for another hour, but I glimpsed at my watch anyway, just to make sure. I began to stare, and my mind dropped into a relaxed Alpha state from the rational, active, thinking Beta state that had me alert and stressed. The Alpha state, I had learned at OHI, was a healing state in which the brain slowed down and was able to absorb new information, become more resourceful, and opened to new possibilities. Twenty minutes later, I was done.

I finished my solar healing and took a two-mile walk on the bike path to the Santa Monica pier and back. I hoped that starting my day immersed in healing would have benefits when I shifted more of my focus to work. I finished my beach time with three sets of ten pushups. I followed each set with ten look-behinds, an exercise I began at OHI to stretch my neck that seemed to help clear up the last remaining fuzziness in my vision.

The minor blurriness didn't interfere with any activity I did as I moved through my day, so the exercise might have been superfluous, but I did it anyway. I wanted the sensation gone. In the three months since I'd started the neck stretch, I noticed less stiffness and greater range of motion. I didn't know whether the stretch was the reason for my improvement, but I didn't want to stop doing it and take a chance.

I returned from the beach and continued my morning routine. I read a passage from *Inner Peace*, repeated my daily affirmations, and made breakfast. I had received a smoothie recipe from a woman at a local raw food store that was loaded with vitamins and nutrients. It contained the meat and milk of a young Thai coconut that I split myself, almond milk, cacao (bitter raw chocolate from the Amazon), almond butter, and maca, a powdered root vegetable from high in the Andes.

I mixed all of the ingredients in a high-powered blender and poured it into a tall glass. It was 100% raw, probably had 700 calories, and most importantly, tasted great. It was a satisfying way to start my day, and I hoped it would help me gain weight. I finished my routine and went to work farming. I set up my growing racks outside our back porch and planted my first batch of wheatgrass. The seeds sprouted by Wednesday. Things were good. My juice bar dream thrived—at least in my imagination.

I wondered what the Nantucket Nectar guys might think of my enterprise. Probably not a whole lot, because by Saturday, I had a problem.

In addition to the half-inch sprouts, the flats were overgrown with white tufts of fuzz. It looked like a sheet of cheesecloth had been dragged across the sprouts and had left behind small clumps of cotton. I remembered from class at OHI that the white puffy stuff wasn't anything nearly as innocuous as cotton, it was much worse—it was mold.

I threw out the diseased tray, scrubbed it clean, and planted a new batch. This time I took the growing rack inside and put it on the kitchen counter. I hoped there was less moisture in the house and that this batch wasn't destined for the trash can, too.

When Robyn got home, I told her all about my situation. She found humor in what had happened, until she looked around the kitchen seeing the "junky" wheatgrass tray in the middle of the counter.

"You're going to move that outside, right?"

"Actually, I was thinking about moving the growing rack that holds the four trays inside, too. There's less moisture in here, and I think that will take care of my mold problem. Can you help me find a good spot in the dining room to put it?"

She paused to let what I'd said sink in. I wanted my wheatgrass flats and cheap-looking growing rack made of plastic piping to "junk up" our remodeled kitchen that she had already retrofitted to our new raw lifestyle. She let me have it.

"You've got to be kidding me! The money you're spending to grow this stuff is more than you would spend to buy a full grown tray of grass from the Co-op. You're smarter than this."

I was conflicted. I didn't want to give up on growing wheatgrass because I didn't want to lose my connection with the cycle of life that had been so integral to my healing. Fortunately, Robyn allowed me to keep the freshly planted growing tray indoors for another run. What I really needed was a vegetable garden to ground myself to the earth.

◆

With one week left before I returned to Sapient, I turned my attention to Robyn. I'd missed her while we'd been apart and because my health had been in decline ever since we'd been married, I didn't feel that I'd been her husband. I felt more like her sick friend. Robyn had assumed many of the responsibilities that most married couples shared, like taking out the trash, paying bills, washing dishes, and doing laundry. Now that I'd regained my health, I'd looked forward to playing a bigger role.

Since I was home for good, we resumed our discussion about starting a family; Robyn's fears surfaced about having a healthy baby. The realities of our circumstance hit her hard. She was almost thirty-five, and she was concerned about the condition of her eggs and the potential for birth defects. She also worried about my genetic makeup and the possibility of our child inheriting my MS.

Our conversation was much more intense than our discussion that merely broached the subject two weeks earlier. Robyn referenced a discussion we had had during a previous neurological exam. She had raised the question about the chance of passing the MS gene onto our child. Andy said there was less than a 4% chance. Robyn didn't react favorably to his explanation. She'd heard too many stories of people with MS having parents who had the disease, and the thought of carrying that life-long guilt made her question getting pregnant.

She suggested that we might want to consider adoption instead, something I had already agreed to early in our relationship, when she first brought it up. There was no way I was going to renege on my word after everything she'd done to stay by my side, but I told her the truth about how I felt now: I wanted us to try getting pregnant. It was my first choice for starting a family, and she agreed.

◆

I wanted to do just about anything to ensure we could raise a child and maintain our comfortable lifestyle. During my four months at OHI, Robyn had taken over the responsibility of paying the bills, which freed my mind from financial concerns, so I could focus on my health. My experience at the institute had challenged my beliefs about many things, including the idea that my value as a person was based on my financial worth, but regardless of my beliefs about money, I needed to find some way to keep a roof over our heads and food on the table.

Since I had returned home, I had a lot of free time and let my mind chase random career fantasies to make the money needed to support our family. My lack of early success growing wheatgrass showed me this wasn't my destiny. Not by a long shot.

The thought of the beach mansion on Boston's North Shore that I'd seen with my brother shortly after the diagnosis never strayed far from my mind; however, changing my profession didn't exactly make me feel more confident about maintaining our lifestyle of choice. During a conversation with MS at OHI, I realized a career change was in order, but I was too focused on regaining my health to even begin considering such a huge shift.

My job at Sapient provided us a good standard of living. Most financial planners who evaluated our position would have been satisfied that we had a solid financial footing, but I believed we didn't have enough. I wasn't sure how much money we needed; I just knew we needed more. At the same time, I feared that returning to my old job might short-circuit my recovery. I was in a true dilemma.

As the day of my return to Sapient loomed closer, I began to think about how my body might respond to the shift in environment. I wanted to experience fluidity and openness on the job, but I knew that wasn't something most office settings supported. Talking about my experiences over the past four months clearly wasn't water-cooler talk either. I grew concerned about how I would discuss my time in San Diego. I was self-conscious about how others might perceive my experience, and I worried that my very non-traditional approaches would be judged as unacceptable, and worse, reflect poorly on my character and thwart my advancement in the company.

How much could I reveal of what had happened since I had taken my sabbatical? I was obviously not the same person who left Sapient four months earlier. The more I thought about my return, the more I worried that I wouldn't be able to balance my priorities. I feared that my job would consume me and that my health would suffer, so I wouldn't be able to become the husband that I wanted to be and that Robyn deserved—let alone the focused, attentive father I wanted to be someday. My mind was reeling again, and I was drifting far from the inner peace I had experienced at OHI.

My colleagues were conscious people, but we worked within a capitalistic structure, where the most important thing at the end of the day was profit. I understood my colleagues would support my healthy well-balanced lifestyle, until they were forced to decide between health and profit. I had excelled at Sapient because I had put in sixty- to eighty-hour weeks to make sure my projects met their commitments. Unfortunately, I knew that if I wanted to progress in my career, I would have to resume my rigorous schedule, jeopardizing my health and well-being. But the time had come to see if it was possible for me to stay healthy while Robyn and I returned to our old life.

Early one morning, late in my final week before I had to return to work, I completed my morning beach routine and thought about how my life might change in a few short days. I wasn't sure how the priority shift I had made at OHI would play out.

I walked toward the Santa Monica pier and considered Matthew Grace's recovery. The idea that he had retrained his body to run after he'd lost use of his legs filled me with optimism. I had given up on my desire to run again before OHI, but each day that my rebuilt body moved better, my confidence grew. My desire to jog came from a different place than the one that obligated me to compete in marathons, triathlons, and scale 14,000-foot peaks. Curiosity and wonder drove me now. As I felt my body regain strength, balance, and sensation, I knew I would run again, but that morning wasn't the day to try. I wanted to get back and see Robyn before she left for work.

That afternoon, I checked on my second batch of wheatgrass. The grass had sprouted, but so had the mold. I wasn't sure what to do. I thought about how OHI had grown their grass and how it differed from what I'd done. I remembered that every time I walked into the greenhouse at the institute, I was hit by a blast of wind and concluded that the huge fans must have circulated the air to keep mold from growing. I would need to get a fan and see if that solved my problem, but I no longer had time during the week to experiment; I had to return to work.

With less than three days until I returned to Sapient, my grandiose dream of becoming 'the wheatgrass guy of Southern California' looked more and more bleak. I bought the fan the following weekend anyway and made one last attempt to grow another batch indoors but failed again. My farming days had produced only mold. I gave up on my idea and decided to buy wheatgrass from the local health food store. To keep the habit affordable, I would reduce my intake of wheatgrass to two ounces per day, five days a week, versus every day, and see how I fared. Though I tried to remain positive, I had a sinking feeling about this new experiment. Deep inside, my intuition was telling me that my recovery and my job were about to do battle. I'd never thought I would need more courage to return to Sapient than I did to start OHI.

28
RETURNING TO WORK

One week after I'd been back at work, I went to lunch with my boss and mentor, Frank, at an upscale café around the corner from the office. I took a seat and recalled the intense fear I had felt during my early OHI days that I wouldn't be able to return to work and have a professional business lunch ever again.

Before OHI, I slurred my speech, my mind went in circles, and my body was weak and diseased, but that frail and fatigued man was gone. Taking his place was a man neither Frank nor I were sure we knew, but we wanted to give him a chance to excel and regain his status. As we caught up, my thoughts were coherent and fluid, rolling off my tongue without distortion or delay. It was clear I was in a different place.

Frank and I had built a trusting relationship working together the previous eight years, and it was easy to get to the heart of my OHI experience. I shared how I'd rid my body of disease, how I'd rebuilt myself through raw food, detoxification, and exercise, combined with the emotional work I'd done to challenge and change my beliefs.

Frank was impressed with my improvement and referenced the light bulb speech I'd made the previous January. I was relieved to no longer live that sickly existence, and we laughed at the old image of me struggling—not because it was funny, but because it was ironic. It was hard for both of us to believe that was me.

I got back to my desk after lunch and reflected on our time together. There was nothing said during our conversation that caused me to become concerned about my professional future. There were no ultimatums about needing to get staffed to a project right away or discussion about how my leave impacted my standing and reputation at the company. I was left with the impression that I had time to find my place again.

After my first month back at Sapient, my mind was clear, my body nimble, and it felt good to be back. I decided to retake the project management course that I'd bombed six months earlier. I finished reviewing the material and eagerly went on to the test, immediately aware that something was different.

Instead of feeling my mind spiral as it tried to grasp concepts, it felt sharp and lucid. The questions and answers made sense. I felt relieved to finish, then hit the submit button and went to the bathroom.

When I returned, I searched the screen for my score. A rush of adrenalin surged through me when I saw that I had earned a 93. I didn't just squeak by, I passed with flying colors. I sat at my desk in silence and stared at the screen. Here was proof that I had regained my mental faculties.

Later that month, I woke one morning full of energy. I completed three sets of fifty bounces on the trampoline, my daily regimen since my time at OHI. I bounded off and steadied myself. I felt the most stable since I'd begun my recovery.

I drank a glass of water and headed to the beach. When I arrived in the parking lot, the sky was overcast—not ideal conditions to sun gaze. Rather than wallow, I walked toward the sand and thought of other ways to get the "chi" energy to flow inside me. My body yearned to feel that tingling, euphoric sensation before I entered the office.

I reached the bike path and considered running. I remembered Matthew Grace's account of learning to run again. He said it was a process that began with walking and involved failing and falling but eventually lead to regaining the ability to run. I was walking well and had even run down the hill at the institute a few times after class, so I knew the day I would once again run along the Pacific was near.

I walked along the bike path in the direction of the Ferris wheel on the pier, about a mile away, and my confidence grew. I picked up my pace and started to stride. I hadn't run more than a few hundred yards in more than two years. I could feel my blood pulsing as I pumped my arms and legs, my lungs had a winded fullness, and I felt relaxed. My "chi" had joined me. I stopped a quarter of the way down the path to re-center myself because I was so excited about what was happening, and I didn't want to risk a fall. After walking a few yards, I resumed my run.

I stopped again to re-center after running another quarter mile. When I reached the pier, I turned around, deciding to walk back to savor the feeling and acknowledge what I had just accomplished. When I reached my Jeep, I climbed in—my body vibrating with excitement. I'd just run the farthest distance since Robyn and I had been in Newfoundland over two years earlier. The euphoria continued during my drive home.

When I returned to the house, I hurried upstairs and into our bedroom to tell Robyn. The sound of the door closing behind me must have woken her because she rubbed the sleep from her eyes as I entered our bedroom.

"I just ran a mile down at the beach!"

"Really! That's awesome."

"I stopped a few times, but it was great."

Robyn sat up in bed. "I know I haven't said much about the changes in your condition over the last five months, but I wouldn't have believed it was possible if I hadn't seen it myself."

"Me either," I said, wondering the extent of this miraculous turnaround.

◆

That fall, Robyn passionately pursued her interest in the curative powers of food. As a vegetarian for the past twenty years, she knew firsthand the connection between food and health. Her conviction about the link crystallized as she witnessed my recovery. She helped me prepare most of my meals and worked to complete her nutrition degree, but as we sat at the table after dinner one night, I could tell something was bothering her. "What's up?" I asked.

"I'm about to finish my associates degree and not sure I want to spend two more years in school."

"Why? Are you concerned about the cost?"

"That's part of it. I'm really excited about the raw cheesecakes. I can see it! They will be about an inch thick with a creamy glaze dripping down the side that you can see through a clear plastic container. There will be a red and orange label on the front."

"Sounds cool. Where will you sell them?"

"Probably natural food stores across LA, like the Co-op and maybe even Whole Foods. If I could get into Whole Foods that would be big!?"

"HUGE! I think you're onto something."

"Really? You do . . . ? I think about it all the time. When I first wake up, all day at work, and it's the last thing that runs through my head before I go to sleep."

"So you're having trouble deciding between finishing your undergraduate degree and starting a cheesecake business?"

"Yep."

"What would you rather do?"

"Cheesecakes, of course, but I don't think that makes sense."

"Why not? You're obviously passionate about it. Just think about it."

"Seriously?" she said.

"Yeah, seriously!"

A few weeks later, she gave her notice at work, stopped pursuing her degree in nutrition, and worked to create the raw vegan cheesecake business. I watched from the sidelines as she feverishly completed the major requirements to start her business, from securing licensing to procuring kitchen space. I was impressed. After a month, the only thing left to figure out was what to call the business.

One afternoon, while Robyn brainstormed ideas with her sister, the name Nude Foods popped into her mind, with the tagline "eat it raw" that her brother-in-law had come up with. The name embodied the product's pure, healthy ingredients and had a playful, sexy appeal. Elated she had found a name, Robyn quickly registered the trademark.

September was busy. I continued to heal and worked to get back in the swing of things at work, while Robyn completed the requirements to start Nude Foods and wrapped up her time at the hair salon. Since we'd decided to start a family, we worked hard and played hard. We enjoyed this special time getting reacquainted. Like the other parts of my body that regained function, my ability to have sex returned. This was probably the most incredible part of my recovery. I didn't need to take a little blue pill before having sex, and the feeling of freedom was incredible. We took it slow and easy, enjoying the harmony of life together.

One morning, we had a rare fall rainstorm. I couldn't sun gaze and would need to spend the better part of my time before work putting the soft-top on my Jeep, so I wouldn't get wet on my way into the office. Robyn spared me the stress and agreed to drive me and pick me up after work instead. On the way home, she ran a red light. It was like the signal wasn't even there.

"Woah! You just ran the light!"

"Oh my gosh! I'm so sorry."

That night, as we prepared to go to sleep, Robyn sat at the end of the bed and read through some papers. She'd been distracted since our drive home. I'd thought about what might be bothering her and became concerned that something might have gone wrong at the kitchen. "Is everything okay with the business?" I asked.

"Everything's fine with Nude Foods, but there's something else."

I assumed she knew that with everything we'd been through, there wasn't anything she could say that I couldn't handle.

"Are you sure you're ready for this?"

I looked her in the eye and nodded.

"Okay . . . I think I'm pregnant."

I replayed the words in my head a few times before I reacted. It was the most earth-shattering news I'd received—bigger than the warning that the Mafia was coming, the MS diagnosis, and Robyn's response to my marriage proposal. I was excited but surprised. Sure, I'd been involved in the act, but after we'd made love a few weeks earlier, I hadn't given it a thought. Now that I was back in Santa Monica, there was more opportunity to connect physically; we were still finding our way back to sex.

I was struck by how oblivious I'd been. My mind raced, and I asked how she'd found out. She said that she'd taken half a dozen home pregnancy tests while I was at work and that they'd all been positive. She had scheduled an appointment with her OB-GYN to have a blood test for tomorrow and wouldn't know for sure for two days.

Two days later, I went to work knowing that Robyn would get a call from her doctor. I would have rather taken the morning off with Robyn to wait for the official news but went to the office instead. I had missed so many days and didn't want people to think I'd gone soft. I just sat and stared at my monitor most of the morning. I was too excited to do anything else. Midmorning, my phone rang.

I didn't have caller ID and answered, "Jon Chandonnet."

"Robyn Chandonnet," she said back, laughing.

"What's up?"

"You're going to be a daddy!"

The line fell silent as I considered the news.

When I hung up, an intense wave of energy surged through me. My dream of being a father was coming true. I felt more alive than ever and even more determined to provide for my family.

In November, Robyn left her job at the salon to launch Nude Foods. I knew the business would be a success because Robyn was highly motivated. The business was strongly aligned with her personal values, it had a million dollar name, and there was a current movement afoot in American culture known as Lifestyles of Health and Sustainability (LOHAS) that said consumers valued socially conscious enterprises and were willing to pay for products that had a positive social impact.

Because Robyn's cheesecakes were made with 100% live, unprocessed ingredients, her business was solidly aligned with the movement. The business held promise to provide a healthy income, but it was new and probably a few years away from yielding anything steady. We just had to make it through the start-up period.

Robyn and I were on the way to realizing our dream of a family, Robyn was on her way to realizing her professional dream, but I felt in limbo professionally. I was grateful that Sapient had welcomed my return because I needed a secure source of income to support our growing family. But after what I'd experienced at OHI, I knew I had a lot more to offer the world than helping others use technology to solve problems; I just wasn't sure exactly what that purpose was.

That fall, I received two tickets to attend a free seminar on building financial wealth featuring T. Harv Eker, author of the book *Secrets of the Millionaire Mind*. I assumed I had received them because I'd bought the book back in July. Whatever the reason, the invite arrived in my mailbox; I found it serendipitous. It was exactly what I needed. At least that's what my rational, conscious mind concluded. I clung to the belief that money was the key to my happiness because I hadn't found another way to align my purpose with my passion and satisfy my needs for food, shelter, and security. I wasn't sure why I had been placed on earth at this time and in this body. I just knew I had to be a healthy partner for Robyn and a father who could provide for our child.

I invited Pete and was pleased he wanted to attend so that I could begin to repay the debt I felt I owed him for turning me on to OHI. Obviously, I had not let go of my need to keep score. Just as I had held tightly to the idea that money was the key to my happiness, I always felt indebted to others.

At the seminar, we learned ways to build wealth through real estate and stock investments. Real estate didn't interest me, but stocks did, particularly a web application known as Investtools. I'd been interested in building financial wealth since I was a ten-year-old searching pockets in the laundry for loose change. I remember one time I found nine one-dollar bills and excitedly exchanged them with my mother for a ten. I was so proud of myself. I had made my first 11% return for twenty minutes of work.

When it was time to find a profession after college, I wanted one that involved building my net worth. I figured I would spend eight to ten hour days working in whatever profession I picked, so I wanted one that afforded me the lifestyle to which I was accustomed. I also was idealistic and wanted whatever I did at work to mean something to others, specifically to improve financial security for low-income families.

I had developed my social conscience during college, where I enjoyed my extra-curricular activities more than my studies. I spent countless hours in pursuit of the goal to create affordable housing through involvement in a campus fundraiser for Habitat for Humanity known as the UR Century. Emboldened by idealism, I put my drive for riches on hold and followed my heart. I took my first job after college working for the Campus Outreach Opportunity League, or COOL, a program funded through President Clinton's newly formed Commission on National and Community Service. I traveled to college campuses throughout the southeastern United States and worked with campus administrators to create sustainable campus-community relationships.

I traveled for two years before I finally decided it was time to get serious about a 'proper' profession, one that would provide the standard of living I wanted. I put my professional passion in the same box as my emotions and went on to graduate school. When I wasn't focused on my studies, I fed my fascination with the stock market. The World Wide Web was just taking off and had lead to the creation of online applications such as Nasdaq.com that I used to evaluate the financial health of a company. In that way, money had become my new passion.

My drive to build wealth kicked in after the diagnosis, but it went into overdrive when Robyn found out she was pregnant. I knew that investing in the stock market was like high stakes gambling, but I knew that I could build wealth through a sound investment approach based on discipline, courage, and conviction—like Warren Buffet and Benjamin Graham said was possible. I greatly admired the investing titans and craved the financial independence they espoused, because I assumed it would bring happiness and the great life I wanted.

It might seem odd that I still defined a great life by my financial wealth, even after I had regained my health, but I couldn't let go of my primal fear of not being able to take care of myself—especially with a child on the way. If I had stopped to slow down, I might have seen that I was already living a great life, but I had more to learn.

Achieving success in the world of investing seemed very similar to the philosophy I had followed to turn my health around. I realized that investing, like healing, could be a certainty if I had the right tools and took a disciplined approach. As I listened to the seminar speakers, I became convinced I could achieve the success I wanted.

I was most impressed by their sophisticated online application and the personal coaching they offered to further improve my chances of success. I paid $10,000 for the online service and a year's worth of coaching. I didn't spend time weighing the pros and cons. I knew it took money to make money and eagerly jumped at the opportunity.

As I drove Pete to the airport after the seminar, he asked if Robyn and I wanted to attend the Falling Awake workshop that he would help to facilitate the following month. The workshop was designed to help people get clear on what they really wanted from life and provided methods to make their dreams a reality. He probably knew that I was searching for a purpose because of my knee-jerk reaction to sign up with Investtools.

I asked Robyn if she wanted to attend Falling Awake with me. I figured it would help me get clear whether or not Investtools was the key to our financial independence. A prior conversation with MS had helped me see that I needed to change my profession if I wanted to tap into my passion. Maybe Investtools was it? If nothing else, the workshop would offer clarity and allow us to create a unified vision for our future.

The day before Robyn and I were scheduled to fly up to San Francisco to 'fall awake,' we packed a cooler full of food for the entire three-day trip because I was still 100% raw, and Robyn was about 50% raw. Pete said there would be a salad bar at lunch and dinner to augment my meals, but I knew I'd need to bring most of what I needed to eat. It was extra work to plan all my meals, but it felt good to know I could maintain my commitment to raw food. Robyn was integral in pulling off the weekend by doing all the shopping and preparing the majority of my meals, watching as I packed the cooler to make sure I didn't forget anything. I could have never done it without her.

It was overcast and rained for most of our stay, but the conditions were ideal for three days of brainstorming and introspection, generating ideas about how to live the life of our dreams. I remember listening to the workshop facilitator, Dave Ellis, and staring out the window, watching rain come down in sheets, when it hit me. My purpose, at least for now, was to make sure Robyn experienced an awesome pregnancy so that our family could enjoy a harmonious start. It was time for me to take on a new kind of leadership.

"I'm going to do everything possible to make that happen," I told her at lunch, realizing she was already way ahead of me on this. Not a day went by that she didn't think about how her actions might impact our baby from driving a car, crossing the street or eating and drinking. "I'm already having an awesome pregnancy," she said and smiled.

As my focus expanded from Investtools to the health of my wife and baby, I grew increasingly annoyed at the workshop's proposition that money didn't need to guide a person's decisions. It was an ironic twist, and clearly a meaningful reflection for the reasons why I had come in the first place. Dave Ellis was a rich man. He had written *Becoming a Master Student*, one of the top selling books on college campuses for years. He was financially set for life and I had difficulty relating to his experience. Once I had a fat bank account through Investtools, I might consider what it meant *not* to allow money to guide my decisions.

During day two, I got past my money hang-up and stumbled upon a totally unexpected outcome—the creation of a personal mission statement. I realized I wanted to be an inspiration for others who faced challenges and to help them create the life of their dreams. The brainstorm began. I could become a professional speaker or write a book about my experience of finding harmony with MS. My head spun I was so excited.

Speaking in front of groups had interested me since college. Moreover, I'd developed public speaking skills through my client work at Sapient. At OHI, I'd become friends with a fellow missionary, a guy named

Jack Barnard, who'd been a speaking coach for over twenty years. I now had reason to get back in touch with him.

I had the interest, experience, and support network to use speaking to tell my story, but writing was a complete unknown. My friend Holly Payne, who I'd climbed Mount Shasta with two and a half years earlier, was the only person I knew who had experience writing professionally. She earned a MFA from University of Southern California and was an acclaimed author, who by that time had already published two novels and whose work had been published in nine countries and six languages.

Holly and I had also worked together during college on UR Century to benefit Habitat for Humanity. She knew I worked hard, and I knew I could count on her; first to be honest about my aspirations and second to trust her with my secret. She didn't know at the time we climbed Shasta that I had been diagnosed, but if I wanted to write a memoir, I was going to have to be comfortable with her knowing about the MS and a whole lot more of my secrets.

When I got home from the workshop, I called her and filled her in on what I'd been up to, and she was impressed with my turn-around. I told her I wanted to write a book about my experience. She encouraged my optimism and said if I wrote a page a day for a year, I'd have a book; at least technically. At the time, I was a solid left-brained, rational thinker and as far from having an active, intuitive right side as a person could be. It sounded easy—all I had to do was write a page per day and I'd reach my goal. Problem solved, right? I was excited to have maybe found my professional purpose, but in doing so, I had no idea what the writing process would demand and how it would change me—again.

That Thanksgiving, Robyn's sister planned a big celebration for both our families at her house in New Hampshire. We hadn't all been together since our wedding a year and a half earlier. We'd told Pete and

Ray the big news of the pregnancy, but kept it secret from our parents. We wanted to successfully make it through the first trimester and to tell them in person. The news was difficult to keep to myself during our weekly phone calls because I was so happy about the prospect of becoming a father.

Soon after my parents arrived in New Hampshire, we sat around the kitchen counter and caught up: Robyn, her sister Raylene, Raylene's husband, Jim, Pete, and both of our parents. I could barely contain myself. Robyn began to speak, and I took her hand.

"We have so much to be thankful for this year," she said. "We bought a house, made major renovations, Jon turned his health around, and I started a new business. I'm not sure we could have accomplished so much without you all."

"You should be very proud of yourselves," her father responded.

"There's one more thing that we need to share."

A look of concern flashed across my mom's face, as if to say, "Oh no, what now?"

"We're pregnant!"

Robyn beamed as she handed out framed pictures of our son's most recent sonogram. We had learned we were going to have a boy and agreed his name would be Jack, a name we both loved.

My mom's look of concern turned to happiness. Her eyes welled with tears and she nearly leapt out of her seat with joy. It was one of the best Thanksgivings we had shared as a family and our future looked bright.

After we returned to California, anxiety overshadowed our excitement. The pregnancy and stress of starting a new business weighed heavily on Robyn's mind; she was also concerned about the several thousand dollars in expenses that she'd spent.

I tried to help her get clear one night while we lay in bed.

"You think it makes sense to move forward with Nude Foods?" I asked.

"I'm not sure. We don't have any orders and I'm not sure if it'll take off."

"Have you followed up with the co-op? I thought they were interested."

"They were, but I haven't heard from them. They probably don't like it."

"Why don't you call tomorrow? They've probably been busy with the holiday."

"I think the best thing to do is call Sarah at the kitchen and tell her I'm giving up my space, so I don't need to pay for another month."

"You sure? Just give the co-op a call."

"No, I think its best I end this crazy fantasy before it's too late! You take the money and invest it."

Before Robyn went to bed, she wrote an email to Sarah at the kitchen saying she wouldn't need her space starting in December. The next day, I went to work. Before lunch, I received a frantic phone call from Robyn.

"I just got off the phone with the co-op, and I'm not sure what I'm going to do."

"What's up?"

"The deli manager loved the cheesecakes. They want everything I can get them as soon as possible!"

"What's this mean?"

"I guess we're back in business!"

29
PREPARING FOR FATHERHOOD

At the start of the New Year, we went to the doctor to check on Jack. I held Robyn's hand and fixated on the grey monochrome image on the sonogram monitor, seeing Jack's head, hands, and feet for the first time. We watched him wiggle and kick. When he extended his little fingers, I wanted to reach out and touch them to reassure him that his dad was here and he wasn't alone; when the doctor turned up the volume on the monitor, and we heard Jack's heartbeat for the first time. I stood mesmerized, listening to the thump-thump of the muscle that circulated life through his tiny body.

Listening to Jack's heart beat for the first time summoned a need deep inside my core to provide for our family. I immediately looked for opportunities to practice the project management, team leadership, and client problem-solving skills that I'd built my career around. I needed to dive back in and quickly. I desperately needed to find a way to integrate my professional and private lives so that my family would thrive. I wasn't sure what that looked like, or if it was even possible to achieve, but I had to *do something*.

As I set out to reassert myself professionally, my parents shared the news that they, too, had made a significant change. They had finally come to accept that Pete and I were permanent California residents. They had given up on the idea that we might return east to raise our families. They wanted to be closer and had started to look for a house in Solvang, a small town in the hills of North Santa Barbara County. If they found a place there, they would only be a two-hour drive away, rather than a six-hour flight. Robyn and I were thrilled that they planned to be closer to play an active role in Jack's life.

As my parents looked for a new house, I was assigned to a project in San Diego and found a way to channel my professional angst. I'd have to travel every Monday and stay through Thursday, but it was an important step in determining if I could continue to heal in a challenging work environment.

Before I left for my first trip, I packed a cooler with raw food for fifteen meals—each breakfast, lunch, and dinner that I would be away. It would be one less thing to worry about while I was on the road. It appeared to be a high-maintenance lifestyle, but at a certain point, I had to just accept that this was my new normal and roll with it.

I woke my first morning on the project intent on continuing my healing regimen. I drank my usual sixteen ounces of water and walked onto the cold, hard concrete of the hotel room deck to sun gaze. Though I wasn't on the beach, I felt the same relaxed, invigorated sense of balance. I was pleased to be able to continue my morning routine so far from home, fortunate to have a room that allowed me to sun gaze, even though I hadn't requested it. I was happy, too, to find an elliptical machine in the hotel gym and rode it, realizing that if I could continue to heal on the road, I'd have more opportunities to advance my career. Even though I missed Robyn and was bummed we weren't together to experience the excitement of Jack's first kick and the tremendous joy of watching a baby grow inside her, we both understood how important it was for me to stay focused on my job.

By mid-March, my confidence evaporated. I struggled to put together the plan needed to complete the next phase of work. My difficulty wasn't due to the complexity of the task, client demands, or an uncooperative team. I didn't have the focus—or the desire and could no longer muster the energy to work the obsessive hours required to create a plan with the level of detail it needed to succeed. I had lost my drive to be a kick-ass project manager. I just didn't have it in me anymore to jeopardize my health for the sake of my job. I was more and more terrified of a relapse. I was starting to feel a familiar tightness in my neck again and a weakness on my left side when I walked. The symptoms concerned me, and I hoped my regimented lifestyle would stem the tide of progression.

The account creative director came to find me in the team area and took me aside looking for an update on the plan. We walked into an empty room, and I took a seat.

"How's it going?" he asked.

I hesitated not sure what to say.

He picked up on my indecision and forced the point. "I had hoped to see something by now. We're scheduled to begin the implementation on Monday, but I haven't seen the plan; are we all set to begin?"

I turned away and searched for something to say. My delayed silence only emphasized my struggle and the director pushed the point.

"Jon, we really need to get this done. You have been working on it for over a week now. It shouldn't take this long. What do you need?"

I turned back to him and spoke. "I've tried to meet with the different tracks separately so I don't waste people's time, but I think we need to pull everyone together in a room, chunk the work out on post-it notes, and do the planning as a group."

"Well, then let's get to it."

I knew what to do but was resisting. I didn't want to push the team the way I had become hesitant to push myself. I didn't want my colleagues to have to do double the work to help put the plan together. My fears of pushing myself were impacting how I was doing my job. We completed the plan with a group that included each of the track leads as well as the assistance of another project manager, but it was clear I had lost my nerve.

When I returned to the Santa Monica office, I sat down and discussed my recent performance with Frank. I sat across from him at a large table in the conference room where I'd given the light bulb speech a year earlier, feeling the disappointment.

"What happened down in San Diego, Chando?" he opened.

"I'm not sure. I think the travel was more than I could handle." I didn't quite come clean that my health was more important than my career.

"How do you want to move forward?" Frank asked.

Rather than scold me for my irresponsibility, he was giving me a way out, and I appreciated that he allowed *me* to suggest how we might proceed, given my screw up.

I took a deep breath. "Maybe there's an opportunity with a project based out of LA that would allow me to get back into the swing of managing a project without the distractions of being on the road."

Frank nodded. "I think there might be an opportunity with your old buddies down in Torrance. There's a small project in the works that might be a good fit."

I liked the idea. I had managed a number of teams and successfully delivered several projects for the automotive client. "Thanks, Frank. I'll knock this project out of the park."

"No need to knock it out of the park, just do a good job."

As I walked out of the conference room, I let out a big exhale. Though I had kept my health concerns from my boss, I was still worried that my recent performance might affect my career. Other than the project management test I had failed when my mind was clouded, professional failure was still new to me.

A week later, I received word from Frank that the project was moving forward and that I was going to lead it. The work wasn't scheduled to begin for a few weeks, so I had time to brush up on the new project-delivery methodology, introduced while I was on leave the previous year. I hadn't spent time learning it because I hadn't fully recommitted to my job, but after speaking with Frank, it might be my last chance.

Prior to the OHI experience, I had always been hesitant to arrive at the office after eight, and I never left before six. During the downtime before my new project started, I didn't need to be at my desk until nine and was able to leave the office by five because I didn't manage a team and didn't need to set an example for others. I only needed to manage myself and relished the chance to get back on track with my healing.

I made the most of the opportunity and renewed my morning routine. I spent an hour at the beach, where I would sun gaze and then walk or run two miles to the pier and back and then return home to write in my journal and read my daily affirmations.

At night, I re-engaged with the Investtools courses that I had put on hold while I worked in San Diego. It felt good to continue my investor education. Studying provided a much-needed professional spark and led me to reconsider a career change to full-time investing, since sometime in the near future, I would have to figure out a different way to make the same amount of income I earned at Sapient. In spite of the upcoming project, somewhere in the back of my mind, I knew my days were numbered.

On April 10, 2006, I celebrated my first full year of being raw. Robyn and I sat down to enjoy the raw meal she had prepared to celebrate. It was a delicious way to celebrate everything we had accomplished and overcome the previous year and everything that awaited us in the new one: the arrival of Jack, the growth of Nude Foods and my parents' permanent move to California.

Despite all these blessings, I could not bear to tell Robyn how I continued to struggle to find my place at Sapient and how I questioned whether Investtools truly provided the spark I needed to engage my passions. I had made a good return in the paper trading account I had set up to practice the concepts, but I had a problem. Capitalizing on the up and down movements of the market on a daily basis didn't hold my interest.

The investing tools had lost their intrigue, and I wasn't sure what, if anything, would engage my professional interest. I didn't know how to talk about my professional angst. My identity was too wrapped up in my job with Sapient, and I didn't want to introduce turmoil into our relationship, especially at a time when things looked so hopeful. But Robyn was having her own internal conflicts. She questioned whether the current mainstream approach to childbirth made sense after comparing stories of friends who had had cold "medical" birthing experiences, versus warm, spirit-centered labor. Since our time at OHI, we had adopted many nontraditional approaches to healthy living and were open to finding a birth option that aligned with our new perspective.

Robyn used the same passion to research birthing that she had employed to start Nude Foods; she relied on her intuition, street smarts, and stayed open to alternatives. She didn't reject the benefits of Western medicine during her pregnancy. She embraced diagnostic testing like sonograms but was leery of the medical procedures commonly used for labor. She wanted Jack to have a more natural and nurturing birthing experience.

She discovered a newly emerging group of professional birthing coaches, known as doulas, whose job it was to make sure that the birth, from the last trimester through delivery, was as spiritually centered as possible. We liked that the doula worked with us and the hospital staff using alternative tools, such as hypnosis (versus pain medication), that allowed women to stay connected to their body during labor and manage the intense sensations. Robyn had benefited from hypnosis during our first weeks together at OHI and believed that working with a doula would allow her to have the birth she wanted.

She found a doula in our neighborhood named Ramona, and at the beginning of May, we enrolled in her eight-week birthing class. The cornerstone of the class was to use hypnosis to transport Robyn into an altered state that would enable her to have a spiritually centered experience.

We spent May and June preparing for Jack. Robyn purchased a refrigerator and freezer to stockpile a month's worth of cheesecakes, so that she could continue making deliveries to the eight stores that consistently ordered cakes. I fully embraced my role as Robyn's birthing coach. Three or four nights a week, we practiced hypnosis scripts. As I read to her in a calm, melodic voice, she would inevitably slip into a deep state of relaxation and drift off to sleep. This special time together strengthened our bond.

I was fortunate I didn't have to confront my professional purpose as we prepared for Jack's arrival. My job at Sapient was focused but routine. I worked with a strong team of Sapient veterans for a former client. The work was familiar and not too stressful and allowed me to maintain my focus on healing and the birth.

Two weeks before Robyn's due date, we treated ourselves to a massage at our favorite Santa Monica spa as a last hurrah before Jack's arrival. After my massage, I felt like a bowl of Jell-O and enjoyed relaxing in the spa, but when I went to get into the shower, my feet slipped out from under me and my right hip slammed hard onto the floor.

As I lay there, I was reminded of my fall down the stairs eighteen months earlier. This time, my right hip throbbed, but I wasn't too concerned. The hip seemed to be my only injury; however, when I placed weight on my right leg, I was overcome by pain and realized there might be more damage to the hip than I thought. Something was definitely wrong. I hobbled to the front desk, wrote out an incident report and asked them to get Robyn.

When I saw her, I lowered my head and told her that I had fallen in the bathroom and was in a lot of pain. She was two weeks from her due date, and the last thing I wanted was for her to worry about me. She let me lean against her, and as we gingerly made our way to the elevator and to the car, I felt like an idiot as my very pregnant wife held me upright. I should have been the one helping her.

When we arrived at the emergency room, the doors swung open, and a nurse approached. "Are you okay?" she asked as she looked at Robyn.

"Yes, I'm fine. It's my husband who needs help."

I gave the nurse a nod of agreement. I was too embarrassed to speak. I spent the next hour in the emergency room being x-rayed then was sent home with crutches. When I got home, Robyn got me an ice pack, made sure I was comfortable, and brought me dinner in front of the TV. She took a seat next to me and we ate.

"I should be waiting on you," I said, feeling helpless as we watched the news.

"Don't worry," she said and rubbed her bulging belly. "You'll have plenty of time to make up for it."

After my fall at the spa, I went to an orthopedic specialist to understand the extent of my injury. It turned out that I had a hairline fracture of my trochanter, the large club-like bone at the top of my femur that fits like a ball into my hip joint. As long as I kept off my leg, I avoided intense shooting pain. I stayed off my feet and missed a couple days of work while I adjusted to the crutches. I felt awkward taking time off work because, at any moment, I would be out for six weeks on paternity leave.

This was the worst time for me to get hurt—two weeks before Jack's birth. I hoped he would stay inside his plush cocoon until I was off crutches and able to help care for him. Wishful thinking; he would come when he wanted.

I stayed off my leg and used the crutches religiously for the next two weeks, refusing to let my injury deter me from doing what I needed to prevent a relapse. I continued to sun gaze each day, completed as much of my daily routine as the hip would allow, and resumed my daily intake of wheatgrass.

By June 28th, the day of Jack's scheduled arrival, I was off the crutches. I was relieved to have regained mobility, and the urgency to heal immediately had lessened because Robyn's mom, Shirley, had arrived from Newfoundland for four weeks.

We were very fortunate to have her with us. Having Shirley around made me hyper-aware of my deficiencies in housekeeping. I had been raised in a male-dominated home without much awareness or appreciation for household duties. I was very fortunate that my mother took care of so many of my responsibilities, like washing my clothes, cooking dinner, and even doing the dishes. Robyn had assumed most household tasks during our first year of marriage as MS ravaged me, but now that I was healthier and with Jack's arrival right around the corner, I needed to take greater responsibility around the house. I wanted to reduce the burden on Robyn and set a good example for our son.

On July second, the day of our second anniversary, our son was still snug in his mom's belly. That morning we went down to the Santa Monica Farmer's Market with Shirley to celebrate our special day. I had surprised Robyn the day before with a dozen roses, but we didn't plan anything more extravagant. We had passed Jack's due date four days earlier. I couldn't wait to meet him, but secretly hoped he would delay his arrival one more day. I wanted July second to remain our special day and his birthday to be a day all his own.

Robyn started to eat and then felt the first flutter of contractions. We didn't panic but cut lunch short, returned home, and made sure

Robyn was calm and relaxed; after she called the doctor, she decided to stay at home and then called Ramona, the doula, to come to the house.

We read through hypnosis scripts to put Robyn into a deep meditative state for most of the day, and by eight o'clock, Ramona left to work with another mother after Robyn said it would be okay. Ramona had asked if Robyn wanted one of her colleagues to fill in for her, but Robyn declined, feeling comfortable with her mother and me. After Ramona left, a rush of anxiety hit me. I had been assigned the most important job of my life: the quality of Robyn's birth was completely up to us. We wanted to make it great.

Two hours later, by ten that night, the contractions had increased significantly and were coming faster; time to go to the hospital. We called my parents so they could drive down and join us and took off.

As I drove, I had visions of husbands rushing around frantically, tending to their pregnant wives. Even though I felt anxious, I didn't rush. As a result of being in a deep state of relaxation after reading hypnosis scripts and moving mindfully due to the hip injury, I remained calm. Once we got to the hospital, I handed over Robyn's birth plan, only to learn after the nurse examined Robyn that she was only dilated two centimeters.

After two hours sitting around with my parents and her mom, Robyn finally hit the wall. Jack wasn't coming anytime soon, and so our parents returned to our house to sleep. The next morning, we were surprised to discover there had been no change in her dilation. The hypnosis we had used to relax her that night had stopped the contractions all together, but they restarted later that morning. Since she had been in pre-labor for twenty-four hours, the doctor gave us the option of staying the course or asked if she could break Robyn's water, in the hope that it would help move the baby along. At first Robyn was hesitant. Though the contractions had been active for the previous twenty-four hours, she still wanted to have as natural a birth as possible.

After carefully considering her options, Robyn decided to go with the doctor's suggestion; she was tired and wanted to meet Jack. The doctor broke her water, and in so doing, compromised the integrity of the womb, increasing the potential for a serious complication. This was a risk we understood, but we took it and started the 24 hour countdown for Jack's birth.

By 10:00 Monday night, half of the safety window had elapsed since her amniotic sac had been broken; Robyn's anxiousness got the best of her. She confided in me that she had had enough after thirty-six hours. "I'm so tired and I'm not sure I have the strength or stamina to push during labor. I think I should get an epidural. I need a break."

Ramona had rejoined us after the other mom had given birth. She stood next to me and gave a nod of agreement. I watched Robyn's eyes well with tears and knew that this wasn't the way she wanted the birth to go. Life had thrown us another curve ball, and we had to find the best way to respond in the moment. We ordered the epidural, and while the drugs went to work, I read her another hypnosis script and she slept soundly until 4:30 the next morning, when the epidural wore off. It was Tuesday, July fourth.

The nurse had called the anesthesiologist to give Robyn another shot, but when he arrived, we found out he wouldn't be able to administer more pain relief. Jack had traveled too far down the birth canal; there was no way to alleviate the pain.

The nurse checked Robyn and saw that her uterus had completely dilated while she had slept. The delivery nurse and I moved into position and coached Robyn through four hours of intense pushing. As the action intensified, the OBGYN arrived on the scene and asked Robyn how she felt. "Just get him OUT!" she pleaded.

The delivery nurse contorted herself into a crazy array of positions to help move Jack through the birth canal. At one point she stood up on the bed frame and struggled to get leverage, while encouraging Robyn and yelling, "PUSH!"

Robyn gave one final hard push, and I watched Jack's cone-shaped head burst through the birth canal. I caught the look on Jack's face as he saw the world for the first time. "Where am I and who are you people?!" Then he wailed. I looked over at Robyn as tears streamed down her cheeks and watched as she reached out to hold her boy.

"Not yet," the nurse responded. He needed to be examined by a pediatric respiratory specialist to make sure he hadn't swallowed any meconium during the delivery. After what seemed an eternity, the doctor finished and handed Jack to Robyn.

I sat in a chair at the foot of Robyn's bed and looked back in awe at the marathon delivery. I was so thankful it ended happily, but I was concerned for Robyn. She had had a forty-eight-hour delivery and had suffered a third-degree tear. I was tired but hadn't pushed a baby out of my body, so I couldn't begin to imagine how physically exhausted she must have been. It made every marathon, the climb up Mount Shasta, and the long day I lost my bike in the Sierras all seem trivial in comparison.

We brought Jack home from the hospital two days later. We walked into the house and set the baby carrier down on the kitchen table. I looked at Jack. He had Robyn's blue eyes and complexion, but he had my hands, feet, and ears. He weighed seven pounds six ounces and was twenty and a half inches long. He was very alert, and his eyes lit up whenever we looked at him. I stared at our perfect baby boy and smiled. This was what it meant to live a great life—to find love and have hope for the future.

I loved that Jack had been born on the fourth of July. Now every year, cities across the country would celebrate his birth with fireworks. I hoped he believed this was true, for his first years anyway. I liked to think that Jack had chosen Independence Day as his birthday to symbolize his father's freedom from disease.

30

REBIRTH

I spent the first two weeks of Jack's life at home with Robyn, Jack, and Shirley, learning "on the job" what it meant to be a new father: help where I could and make sure Robyn felt supported. Jack was doing well, sleeping soundly and gaining weight. We couldn't have asked for a healthier baby, though I felt uneasy about leaving him for a week long writing retreat so soon after his birth. However, with Shirley in town, I was confident Robyn and Jack were in good hands. Robyn had fully supported my decision and even helped prepare the raw food I would need for the week at Skywriter Ranch, the annual summer writing retreat in Crested Butte founded by my friend Holly Payne.

I had always loved Colorado. My brother had lived there and worked as a NOLS instructor, but there was something else about the setting that called me to the writing retreat. Right after Holly had graduated from UR, she was struck by a drunk driver in Crested Butte. It was a very transformative place for her and rather than associate it with the tragedy, she said it was a place of great healing, which strongly appealed to me.

I flew to Colorado and finally arrived at an old mining town Gothic, which since its glory days in the late 19th century, had grown into "RMBL", Rocky Mountain Biological Laboratory, a research station for ecologists and biologists (where Nabokov, a lepidopterist, was rumored to have written parts of *Lolita*). Accommodations were very rustic. I slept in a cabin and used an outhouse: an ideal setting to write. I had brought an eight by eleven picture of Jack, taken a few minutes after he was born, and looked at it first thing in the morning and before I fell asleep each night for inspiration as I sought to discover whether I was truly called to write.

On the second morning, I walked out the front door of my cabin to breathe in the crisp, fresh mountain air at 9,000 feet above sea level. I stood and savored the moment, when a magpie flew up and landed on my shoulder. I had never experienced such an amazing natural occurrence. I had approached many birds before, but every time I got within a few feet, they always flew off. That morning, the visitor came to me unsolicited.

At breakfast, I told my fellow writers about the magpie and someone at the table told me about a Native American proverb: if a magpie lands on you, change is afoot. Apparently, the birds also symbolize creative communication, trickery, the intellect, and in Chinese, good luck. Before OHI, I would have laughed off the bizarre incident as a fluke, but now I trusted that it was not random. The visiting magpie turned out to be an omen of major changes to come that week.

On Wednesday morning, after we had been living at 9,000 feet for three days and my body had adjusted to the altitude, Holly announced that our morning class would be held at a special place, Judd Falls—a majestic mountain waterfall 'not far' from our cabins. She had been teaching us about story structure and the midpoint of every story, reminding us that we were also midway through the retreat. I was taken aback. I wasn't surprised about the excursion—she had alerted us upon arrival, I couldn't believe the workshop was halfway done. I was learning so much and didn't want it to end.

I had mixed emotions about the hike, partly disappointed that all this would be over, but also excited about the four-mile roundtrip journey to an elevation higher than 10,000 feet. I was curious and apprehensive to see how my body would react, given the last mountain I had climbed was Shasta. The hike was shorter than my previous mountain excursions, but it would be a good test of how far my rebuilt body would carry me.

Holly said the hike was moderately strenuous, but not to worry. If I couldn't keep up, the group would wait. I could take all the time I needed, she said, though I hated the idea that I might slow the group— just like I had on Shasta. This time, I didn't allow my ego to drive me. Instead, I followed my curiosity and sense of wonder as I had done during my first morning run to the Pier after my return from OHI. I wanted to reach the waterfall and I craved the sense of accomplishment I'd felt on previous climbs.

I left my cabin to join the others walking down the access road, and we noticed a huge 'S' had been formed by a cloud in the bright blue sky. We all stopped to take a picture. Clearly, something was guiding 'the Skywriters' as we called ourselves that week. I took it to mean that I was right where I needed to be.

After walking a third of a mile across the graded fire road, we reached the trail. I was pleased that my body had moved easily over the smooth road, but the moment we started up the hill, I realized this wasn't going to be easy. As I scrambled up the loose rocks and gravel, I began to feel the effects of the route; the altitude, the steepness of the climb, and my pace conspired to throw me off balance.

I slowed down and deliberately focused on my breathing. The old "Chando" would have pushed the limits and stumbled—unwilling to show any signs of fatigue. However, my time at OHI had taught me to dwell comfortably within myself, so I slowed and followed my body's natural rhythm.

We gained a few more hundred feet of elevation, and I traveled comfortably within my own limits. When we reached the three-quarter mark of the trip, I began to struggle. I hadn't conditioned my legs to climb since I turned my health around, so they had lost the strength to carry me uphill. I asked the group to stop, so I could rest. As we stood and chatted, Brent, one of the guys in our group, made a recommendation.

"I think walking sticks would make things easier."

I knew from my time in the mountains that walking sticks would allow me to use my arms to propel myself more easily uphill.

"Good idea," I said.

Brent, along with Helge, another guy in our group, jumped into the woods to find sticks. They returned each holding a stripped-down Aspen branch for me to use.

"Those will work," I said and jabbed each into the dirt.

Armed with walking sticks, I was able to step up my pace and make good time. I became lost in the cadence of my breathing until I heard the loud crash of water on rocks. A few moments later, I found myself standing on the edge of a rock outcropping, looking at water crashing through a gorge several hundred feet below. I had reached my destination, and a wave of euphoria engulfed me.

I looked over at Brent and Helge and, with sincere gratitude, told them how much I appreciated their help. Before my time at OHI, I was blinded by foolish pride and never would have accepted assistance of any kind, but I'd left the weight of my ego, along with those twenty-five pounds, behind in San Diego.

For the rest of the morning, Holly conducted class overlooking the gorge. When we returned to camp, the descent was naturally much easier than the climb. The final two days of the workshop flew by as I immersed myself in the relaxed, intuitive environment that allowed me to create and thrive.

On Friday night, we went into town for dinner to celebrate. Just before we arrived, there had been a late-afternoon thundershower and when we got to town, we saw the most vibrant double rainbow arched across the sky. I had never seen a rainbow as huge and as bright as this one. All the signs were adding up: the visiting magpie, the "S" in the sky, the hike and now this spectacular light show spoke deeply to my soul. I was on the right path, even if, on occasion, I needed walking sticks to travel it.

After Skywriter Ranch, I went back to work and remained focused on my health. While Jack continued to grow, so did my daily sun gazing ritual. I went to the beach every day upon waking. One morning, before I got out of bed, I watched Jack stretch his arms and legs next to his mom, and I saw Robyn stir. Light had just begun to stream through our window and I had only a few minutes until I lost my opportunity to sun gaze.

"I'm going down to the beach and will be back in an hour," I whispered to Robyn.

I knew this healing technique still didn't sit well with her, so I spared her the details. I was disappointed that we didn't discuss things beyond that, but I realized early in our relationship that we didn't need to agree on everything.

Robyn looked up at me and said, "Could you stay home this morning? I was up a lot last night with Jack, and I need you to take him downstairs so I can get some sleep."

I stood at the foot of the bed disappointed; I wanted to tell her that I needed to go to the beach to sun gaze and exercise because they were essential to my health, but I held my tongue. I also knew Robyn wouldn't have asked me to stay unless she absolutely needed to rest, so I picked Jack up and carried him downstairs.

Shortly after I held him in my arms, my disappointment faded. While Jack and I sat, smiling and laughing, I considered a permanent change to my morning routine. That hadn't been the first time Robyn had asked me to play with Jack in the morning, and I realized I needed to show more responsibility before work to allow Robyn to sleep. This meant I would need to sun gaze at the end of the day if I wanted to continue the practice.

As I considered how to handle this shift in my routine, Robyn's original fear about my sun gazing resonated more strongly. I was seven weeks away from the forty-five-minute mark and didn't want to chance losing my appetite, what HRN had said might happen. Food had become sacred for us. I liked to sit with Robyn at dinner and discuss our day over a meal. Eating together helped us maintain our connection, so I decided it was time to stop sun gazing and become the father and husband I had hoped to be.

Four weeks after Jack was born, we hired a nanny four days a week so Robyn could go back to work. She had begun to consider ways to grow the business, when she answered an unsolicited call from the Dairy Manager at Whole Foods in Woodland Hills. He called to say he had received a number of requests from customers who wanted Nude Foods cheesecakes. Robyn could hardly believe her good fortune and over the next few weeks, worked out the details to get her cheesecakes on the shelf of the biggest organic and whole food supermarket in the country.

Over the next three and a half years, she would grow the relationship between Nude Foods and Whole Foods to include twenty-two of the twenty-four stores in the LA area. Revenue from Whole Foods was integral to Nude Food's 100% annual growth each of the next three years. During that time, I often marveled about Robyn's Field-of-Dreams-like marketing strategy. *Make it, and they will eat.*

Change was afoot in other ways. By the end of October, I decided to step away from my nine-year career in project management. It wasn't something I initiated. I had received feedback from a team member that my project management skills hadn't met team expectations. My shift in priorities had finally caught up to me.

I spoke with Frank about the feedback, and he again gave me an out. He had just taken over human resources and asked if I was interested in a new challenge—recruiting. I said I was interested, and before I shifted my role within the company, Frank made sure I understood that I would be leaving client-focused projects—the most highly esteemed work at Sapient. I didn't mind the change in status. It meant less stress, held the promise to bring greater life balance, and most importantly, prolonged my employment.

"I look forward to the challenge," I said.

It seemed too easy to make the switch, and I was suspicious about why Frank offered me the out. I secretly wondered if state or federal regulations required him to make accommodations for people with health conditions. Offering me another, less risky, job in the company would have been much easier than asking me to leave.

My imagination ran wild and left me feeling uneasy. I began to seriously doubt my worth at the company. I had never asked for special consideration or hinted at the need to be treated differently than my coworkers, but there was no denying that I had an incurable disease and my colleagues were making appropriate adjustments. Whatever the reason, I remained at Sapient for the next year and a half and continued to battle my ego.

31
ROOT CAUSES

Ayear earlier, soon after my return from OHI, I had begun the art of Nei Kung, a slow, deliberate martial art that stimulated my parasympathetic nervous system and was an important part of my healing environment at home. When I began, I told my instructor about my intention to recover from the effects of MS and had diligently attended most Saturday sessions since to bring greater balance into my life. In the twelve months that I had been studying with him, we never talked about my MS, and my teacher respectfully never offered any advice, until one day after class, when he asked how things were going.

I told him my healing seemed to have reached a plateau and that I wanted to go deeper. He mentioned a friend, Jim Emke, who helped people get to the root cause of their MS. He said Jim had more than twenty-five years of experience working with people who had autoimmune disorders. Jim lived in Hawaii but consulted with people over the phone. I was intrigued and asked for his number. I had dramatically improved my health while at OHI but knew some symptoms had resurfaced.

I called Jim, and first asked about his experience. He was a certified nutritionist who had opened an integrated healing clinic in Milwaukee during the mid-seventies. He had extensive experience working with people like me, helping them improve MS conditions. After a successful thirty-year career, he sold the clinic and moved to Hawaii but still consulted with people part-time because of his vast experience and his passion to help people in need. He sounded legitimate, so I shared the highlights of my case.

I provided details of my turn-around spurred by my detox and raw lifestyle, but told him my recovery had seemed to plateau if not regress. I felt unbalanced. My right side was much stronger than my left, which was most noticeable every time I took a step, but also clearly evident when Andy tested my arm and leg strength during neurological exams. I also had a stiffness in the joint where my neck attached to my spine. It felt like sand had gotten stuck in there, and though I had exercised almost every day over the previous year, I lacked the stamina I once knew and tired much more easily as I went through my day.

Jim asked about my health history. I told him I had mono at sixteen, a spell of phantom fatigue at nineteen, and then spoke about the optic neuritis and the incident on the basketball court that led to the diagnosis.

Curiously, Jim then inquired about my dental history.

"Why?" I asked. I had never considered a link between my mouth and MS. Jim said he'd seen a connection between MS and people who had had mercury fillings and root canals during his career at his Milwaukee clinic. I said I didn't have any fillings, but told him that my two front teeth had undergone root canals as the result of an accident on the basketball court in high school.

I was curious how MS and dental work were related. Jim said fillings were often forged from mercury, which was a neurotoxin, and could contribute to the onset of the disease. He also said root canals had the potential to cause a chronic infection that might trigger MS. He then mentioned he used blood work as well as hair and stool samples to better understand whether an external factor might have contributed to someone's condition. He asked if I wanted to work with him to see if my body still harbored an infection or toxin that might be impacting my health. I agreed. I had nothing to loose.

I hung up, encouraged but still skeptical. All my prior doctors had only treated MS symptoms but hadn't considered potential root causes. This was the key difference between Western, allopathic medicine and a more naturopathic approach to treating chronic illness. Jim's test kit arrived. I had blood drawn, collected hair and stool samples, and sent them off for evaluation.

A month later, I received ten pages of results. At first glance, nothing seemed out of the ordinary. I hadn't been trained to understand the numbers, so I sent them to Jim and scheduled a call. He said things looked normal for the most part. I didn't have heavy metal buildup in my tissues, my blood pressure and cholesterol continued to be excellent, and the ratios of vital metabolic minerals were all within expected ranges, but there were two results that raised concern.

My level of vitamin D and white blood cell count were both considerably below normal. Jim said vitamin D was vital to numerous body systems, including the manufacture of nerve cells and the transmission of neural signals. This was significant because MS was essentially a neurological disorder. He said I could easily increase my levels by taking a supplement—or through frequent sun exposure.

My mind jumped to sun gazing. I had spent the previous year staring at the sun and had reached thirty-eight minutes of consecutive gazing per day. Shouldn't that have satisfied my sun exposure requirements? I considered my experience. I had diligently avoided ultraviolet radiation, so I didn't damage my eyes. I knew my body couldn't produce Vitamin D without UV rays, so I realized sun gazing wouldn't have increased my Vitamin D levels. Jim's recommendation was a good one. I made a note to pick up supplements and spend more time outdoors exposing myself to the sun's UV rays.

Jim made another suggestion based on my dental history and low white blood cell count. He said I might want to get a full x-ray of my jaw to rule out an infection. I questioned this and told him I had regular x-rays when I had my teeth cleaned. He told me these wouldn't help because the typical x-ray stopped a few centimeters above the gum line.

I needed one that looked deep into the bones of my mouth and jaw to see if there might be an infection at the end of either root-canalled tooth.

A few weeks later, I had a black and white scan of my jaw that showed a dark region above my number nine tooth that was consistent with bone loss and might be the result of an infection. The root had been removed twenty-three years earlier after the accident on the basketball court. The visible part of my tooth, above the gum, had remained in my mouth for another six years, until it was knocked out on the lacrosse field. The stub of the root canalled tooth still remained in my mouth as a potential host for bacteria that could have been spreading throughout my body.

It suddenly struck me that the infection might have been present in my mouth, wreaking havoc on my health, for more than *twenty years*. MS might not have been the result of 'chance' after all. I had learned at OHI that if my body was filled with the right things—food, water, thoughts, and emotions, it could find its way back to health, but since my symptoms lingered—the fatigue, lack of strength on my left side, absence of synchronicity between the left and right sides of my body, I couldn't help but think there was some deep-rooted structural issue in my body, like an infection.

Was my MS the result of a number of factors that conspired against my body to allow multiple sclerosis to take root? I wondered if my body's apparent difficulty in assimilating vitamin D, my wheat, dairy, and processed food diet, the root-canalled teeth, the stress I put myself through, and my lack of emotional expression were the biggest culprits. I had taken action to address each except the teeth and was encouraged that I might be on the trail of another culprit. I would never know for sure which, if any, of these factors had contributed to my condition, but I was encouraged by the results of the x-ray. However, I wanted a second opinion to corroborate the findings. Another trusted dentist in Los Angeles confirmed the result, and I excitedly called Jim.

My enthusiasm quickly turned to anxiety when Jim gave me my options: I could have an apicoectomy, where an oral surgeon seals off the broken root and removes only the infected soft tissue, or undergo a more radical procedure that would extract what remained of the two old dead teeth, the part below the gum, and clean out the potentially diseased bone that had held the stub tooth in place.

The second option sounded extreme, and I asked Jim to elaborate. He said the most effective way to deal with infections that had reached bone was to clean out the tooth socket, cut away the layer of bone surrounding the diseased teeth, and remove the periodontal ligament, a procedure know as cavitation. He stressed that bone infections were difficult to completely get rid of by removing only the diseased soft tissue. He warned that if these kinds of infections were not properly eradicated, they would fester.

I hung up, conflicted—thrilled to hear I could get rid of the infection but uneasy about how. The surgery seemed too radical. Traditionally, I opted for the least medically invasive procedures. I developed this belief as a boy when I had hurt my knee wrestling in the eighth grade. Based on my dad's advice, I chose physical therapy and rest over arthroscopic surgery to fix a damaged ligament. As a result, I went on to play high school and college athletics, compete in marathons and triathlons, rock climb, and mountain bike without any lingering effects. I knew radical surgery wasn't always the best option.

I decided to pursue the less extreme course—to have an oral surgeon seal the cracked root canal and remove just the infected soft tissue, leaving the two dead tooth stubs in my mouth with minimal recovery time and less chance of a complication. I trusted my body's ability to heal itself and believed that if the infected soft tissue was removed, my body would take care of the rest, like it had done at OHI.

Robyn drove me to the oral surgeon's office for the apicoectomy. The doctor gave me a shot of Novocain, and I stared out the window as I waited for it to take effect. I hoped the procedure wouldn't hurt. I'd had oral surgery before and had received local anesthesia to numb the pain, but I had always felt intense throbbing as it wore off.

Surprisingly, this procedure was almost painless. The only uncomfortable part was the occasional sound of scalpel against bone.

When he finished, the doctor told me he had removed a significant infection, and that he would see me in a month to make sure it had healed.

I met Robyn in the waiting room. Before we got into the car she asked to see the stitches, so I lifted my lip.

"OOWWWW, that looks gnarly. It must hurt."

"I can't feel anything because of the Novocain."

When we got home, I went upstairs to sleep. I had taken the rest of the day off because I expected to be sore. Two hours later, I awoke confused. I expected my mouth to throb, but I didn't feel any pain, not even from the stitches. When I went downstairs, Robyn asked how I felt. "Fine," I said.

She looked confused. "There is no way you're not in pain, you must be in denial."

In the days following the surgery, I didn't feel any differently; I only felt a sense of warmth, hoping I had done everything I could to take care of the infected soft tissue.

32

BUILDING MORE STRENGTH

Assuming the infection was gone that spring, I focused on building a stronger body. I had a solid foundation for health but hadn't gained any weight, hovering at 140 pounds for the previous two years. I wanted to pack on pounds and build muscle and had tried a full spectrum of raw foods, but I hadn't gotten any bigger. I was hesitant to alter my regimen but wanted to see what was available and kept an open mind.

I took a look at what was out there and came across *The Maker's Diet* by Jordan Rubin about improving Crohn's Disease through an all-natural diet that included raw greens, fruits, and vegetables, to which I was accustomed, but also included some cooked meat and grains. Since Crohn's Disease was also an autoimmune disease, I knew the path to recovery might be similar to that of MS.

Through his own natural regimen, Rubin had built muscle mass and put on forty pounds. He built a bigger, stronger body and fully recovered from the effects of his disease. Even though his book was light on scientific studies, it had the proof I most needed. His personal experience showed his regimen worked. *The Maker's Diet* was full of validating insights, like the importance of controlling "the three I's" of illness: infection, inflammation, and insulin; I had heard of these ideas at OHI, but they hadn't crystallized until I started reading more.

I knew from seventh grade science that an infection was the colonization of a foreign organism in the body. In my case, it was probably the bacterial infection in my mouth that I hoped was taken care of. My dental experience reiterated the importance of watching for nasal congestion, lethargy, and fatigue as symptoms of an infection. I concluded that the phantom fatigue I felt at nineteen might not have been such a mystery, but rather the result of my body fighting the infection above my tooth. My body instinctively recognized the signs of infection—I just needed to see them myself.

Inflammation, the second "I", was defined as the body's vascular response to an irritant, such as an infection or other foreign body like a free radical or toxic substance. Inflammation was considered "bad" because it was accompanied by pain or swelling, but it also served to set off alarm bells. The warning system probably hadn't worked for me because the nerves above my two front teeth had been removed during the root canal in high school, so I didn't feel discomfort while the infection raged.

Insulin was the third "I." The key to maintaining a healthy balance of insulin in the blood was to avoid eating foods that raised sugar levels. From my reading at OHI, I knew these foods. They were refined sugars, refined complex carbohydrates, and alcohol. It made complete sense why OHI's meal programs offered two options: foods with limited natural sugar content such as vegetables, or foods with higher sugar content such as fruit. I chose the low sugar diet that I continue to this day.

I also read *Healing Multiple Sclerosis* by Ann Boroch about how Boroch also battled MS with a regimented diet, reworked thoughts, and emotional cleansing. Her routine was similar to mine, but it included cooked foods, like plant-based proteins such as rice and quinoa, as well as lean meats. My research was causing me to re-evaluate my 'raw rule.' My raw, detox lifestyle had allowed me to improve my health, but I wondered if it was the approach I needed to build a stronger body. I questioned how much of the diet I needed to maintain to stay healthy.

I decided to relax my raw rule and experiment with cooked food. I remained about 50% raw, as I slowly introduced proteins to build strength. I had one serving of meat per day, limiting the intake to free-range turkey, an occasional piece of fish, or free-range chicken, and watched for any signs that these foods might trigger any MS symptoms. I made sure the meat didn't contain harmful hormones and fillers, and I stayed away from red meat and pork because of the saturated fat and harmful free radicals. I occasionally ate rice pasta or quinoa to augment my protein and caloric intake.

As I integrated the new teachings, I discovered that Ann Boroch, the author of *Healing Multiple Sclerosis*, was a licensed naturopath who worked with patients in the San Fernando Valley, a twenty-minute drive from my house. I was thrilled that she was so close, and I scheduled an appointment. During our first face-to-face meeting, she hooked me to a biofeedback machine, and I recounted my ten-year odyssey living with the disease. As we spoke, I realized we shared many of the same beliefs about healing.

Before we wrapped up, she handed me a reading of my emotional health during our conversation. The printout showed how I responded emotionally to an external stimulus like a word or concept over the course of our visit. As I sat across from Ann and talked, the biofeedback machine gathered my emotional response to our interaction. The machine took a read on eighty-five emotions; my scores ranged from 48 to 133. Ann drew a line marking the 50 and 100 lines on the graph and explained the printout.

She said an emotion that scored below 50 or above 100 showed my response was unbalanced and merited further examination. I scored 48 in response to my feelings of inadequacy, the only emotion of mine scoring below fifty. I scored above 100 in three emotional areas: feeling misunderstood (103), feeling obsessive (106), and needing variety/feeling bored (106). One emotion was off the charts. My desire to be different hit 133. It was amazing that a one-hour conversation yielded such a comprehensive and accurate view of my emotional health.

Later that night, I gave Ann's findings more consideration. I thought about my scores and brainstormed areas of my life where I wasn't reaching my potential. I knew that I made great strides with my health and that I put all I had into being a husband and father. Two of my top three priorities weren't the source of my stress. I was relieved.

Work, however, continued to present conflict. I knew that while the hiring role at Sapient enabled me to keep a roof over our heads and food on the table, it also had a negative impact on my health because it didn't allow me to live my passion.

No other viable professional option presented itself at the time. I had never before tuned into my feelings of being misunderstood, obsessive, and bored. No wonder these patterns were off the charts. They all had to do with my professional life. Clearly, my career was not aligned with my emotional health. The time had come to face the most terrifying truth I had encountered along my journey with MS. Like it or not, I needed a career change if I ever hoped to improve my health and happiness indefinitely.

33
THE LONG GOOD-BYE

That summer I continued to build confidence in my writing and, again, headed to Colorado to attend Skywriter Ranch. I went to immerse myself in an environment that allowed me to live my dream of telling my story, but I found so much more. By the end of the week, Holly agreed to be my writing coach. I would be the first full-time coaching client Holly had ever taken on, and we were both as excited as we were nervous.

One night in late December of 2007, Robyn and I sat in bed and discussed the great year we'd had—our strengthened relationship, the joy we felt with Jack, Robyn's success with Nude Foods, and my progress with writing. We had accomplished a lot and had many things to be thankful for, but I felt something was missing.

We stayed up and tried to get to the heart of what bothered me. No matter how much balance I had achieved in my life since OHI, we both knew my job caused me to live out of balance and impacted my health. I finally voiced my need to leave Sapient and the security, familiarity, and prosperity of my job. I felt tremendous relief to finally speak the truth that I had known for almost *three years*. Since my second month at OHI, I knew that I had been living out of alignment with my true passion.

"I will support you and any decision that you make," Robyn had told me that night, swallowing the tremendous fear she had about our financial future. We both knew that without my health, our family's prospects for prosperity were bleak at best.

♦

That winter, we put the house on the market and sold or gave away many of the furnishings. We were on a mission to downsize and simplify. Soon after, the housing bubble burst, and the economy plunged into a downward spiral not seen since the Great Depression. We had a young child, a new business, a house on the market, and I was in the midst of a healing journey that demanded I leave my career.

Though we questioned whether we had made the right decision, we realized there was no other choice. My body couldn't handle the daily rigor of corporate life. MS simply refused to allow it. Had I chosen to continue, I would have been lying to myself and ignoring the truths that had eluded me for so long. I couldn't stop now. I was at the point of no return. I wanted to keep walking. I wanted to run on the beach with Jack. The stakes were way too high for me to use denial again to cope.

The only real decision we had to make was exactly *when* I was going to leave Sapient. Robyn's increased sales at Nude Foods and my growing confidence in writing helped us keep the faith. We carried the mortgage and paid rent on the smaller place we planned to move into for three months until we found a buyer for the house. Those were anxious times. I sat awake many nights, wondering what we would do if it didn't sell.

Just when I thought I had a handle on the changes we faced, I received my annual review at work for my previous year's performance. The comments were mostly negative, which didn't surprise me, but they did concern me. In the past, I would have pushed myself beyond my limits to accommodate everything in my life, but not after I had reordered my priorities. Frank scheduled a meeting to discuss the annual review.

"Jon, I assume you've read the feedback?"

"I have, and I discussed it with my manager."

"This isn't what I expected when you took on the role. What's up?"

I let him know how I felt. "I don't think there's a role at Sapient that will allow me to balance my work and health, and I think it's time for me to find a profession that allows me to maintain greater work-life balance."

Frank met my gaze and calmly continued. "It doesn't need to go that way. We may be able to find another place for you. I've done that for a few guys. It only extended their time here for another year, but it might be an option."

"I appreciate the consideration, but I need to make the change for the sake of my health."

I didn't go into the details. Finally, after all this time, I knew that my health included not only my physical well-being, but my emotional well-being, too. I truly appreciated Frank's willingness to accommodate my needs. That was so characteristic of Sapient, and I knew I would miss working with people like him and so many others who had helped me grow over the course of my career. But my real manager was MS now.

That spring, I said good-bye to Sapient. The afternoon of my farewell, I walked into the empty conference room and prepared for my talk. After I organized the chairs, I took a seat and glimpsed at the clock; it was 4:55, five minutes before I was to begin.

I ran through my opening one last time. I was dreading my speech and my body was tense. I breathed shallowly, thinking about the room full of people focused on my every word. Would I be able to connect with the audience? Would I be able to convey the important parts of my story? Would my voice flow smoothly, or would it be strained and broken like during the light bulb speech? Would they fully understand my reasons for leaving such a great company?

Since OHI, I had tried to rid my life of as much stress as possible but realized some stress was good. The stress I felt that afternoon was the good kind. It had me on edge, like a sprinter waiting for the gun to sound. I knew the best way to deliver a message and connect with the audience was to speak from the heart.

Instead of memorizing the speech, which I would have done in the past, I prepared differently. I had made a high-level outline of my five major points and committed them to memory. That was all I did. I hoped this radical departure from my over-prepared and rehearsed style would allow me to connect with the audience.

I took another look at the clock—it was 4:59. With less than sixty seconds to go, no one was in the room. The empty seats were arranged in a circle, and I anxiously moved from one chair to the next, trying to find a comfortable spot, all the while fearing that no one cared I was leaving.

I heard Lu approach and breathed. At least I had one colleague in the audience. I figured Lu and I could leave and have a beer at this point. I was so nervous, I might have taken a sip, even though I hadn't had a drop of alcohol in three years. Lu had come to hear me talk and I welcomed him. He made no comment about the empty chairs but took a seat and waited with me.

It was because of him and Kevin Hughes, my first of four career mentors at the company that I was in this room. I had brought up my exit strategy a few weeks earlier. I told them I would be leaving the company and asked them to keep it confidential. I believed that sneaking out was a much better way to go, but I was only re-enacting the same behavior I'd learned the morning after the woodpile, when my father said it would be best not to tell anyone about my mom. I didn't want my decision to affect office morale. I assumed I would just ease out with as little fanfare as possible. Kevin had told me exactly what he thought about my strategy: it was a shitty idea.

"You know what, Chando? That's the exact wrong thing to do. You're a fixture at Sapient LA and you need to be more up front."

"Really?"

"Fading away like that will have a bigger impact on morale than a more public departure because it will lead people to draw their own conclusions. Let people say good-bye."

I was glad I listened to Kevin and Lu. One by one, more colleagues entered the room. I sat there and watched in gratitude as every chair filled. The circle was complete. Lu glanced over and smiled.

When Frank walked in, I knew it was time. Frank looked over at me and spoke, "I'm not sure if people know this, but I'm pretty sure Chando was the first LA hire."

He went on to tell of my contributions and impact on the office. When he was finished, he asked if anyone else wanted to share a story. For the next fifteen minutes, we heard stories from people who had been with the company anywhere from two to ten years. The theme was the same—I would be remembered for my passion, drive, excitement, and strong impact on the LA office. The stories also highlighted my crazy weekend adventures that often led coworkers to limp to work on Monday with tall tales.

After all of the accolades, my anxiety disappeared, and I thanked everyone for coming, grateful for the things they said. I explained how my world had crashed around me and led me to make a drastic lifestyle change to support my health, so that I could live a great and long life with my wife and son. People remained silent as I spoke about my time at the Optimum Health Institute and how my lifestyle changes had altered the disease's progression and unlocked my body's natural healing powers.

I related how I had been able to heal by living in harmony with MS, and I shared my most profound belief, that MS was essentially a disease of imbalance. I said that I had been a 78 record spinning at 120. I was out of control before I got my body rebalanced through exercise, diet, detoxification, meditation, cleansed emotions, positive thinking, toning, and sun gazing. I told them how the pain dissipated, and then disappeared, the stiffness dissipated, and then disappeared, and how I knew that I was healing.

When I finished my remarks, I opened the room to questions. Hands went up immediately, and I went around the room. One question really stuck with me.

"What was the key to your turn-around?"

"Hope," I said, then added, "I allowed love into my heart and found the courage to face MS. The love for my wife and family enabled me to find the right path and opened my eyes to the healing world—one of faith, whole live food, and the spirit."

I told the group how I failed an online test for a course in project management that I had been at the company long enough to teach. I reminded my colleagues how I had lost feeling in my hands and feet and that my voice had been weak and strained. Several in the room had witnessed this firsthand during the light-bulb speech I had given three and a half years earlier. I watched people in the audience turn to their neighbor and whisper a comment and saw pained expressions flash across faces. I shared how desperate I had become, and eventually how I had lost all hope that I would recover, which culminated in my decision to attend OHI.

When there were no more questions, I thanked everyone for coming and reminded them that I lived down the street and was happy to still be neighbors with Sapient. As I left the parking garage, I realized it was the last time I'd make that trip.

I was heading home to my new life with my wife and my young son. I gripped the wheel and beamed, feeling the Southern California sun on my face. I headed west toward home in the direction of the setting sun, knowing that it was possible to feel the same way I did when I left OHI three years prior.

Later that week, I received an e-mail from Frank. "Wednesday night was a good moment for me. You did a nice job, and I wish you all the best. "That said a lot. Frank was hire number forty, and there were now over six thousand people in the company across the globe. Even though I had left the corporate world, a new job awaited me. I was leaving behind the darkness of the shadow summit to live a vibrant life in harmony with my mind, body, spirit, emotions, and the people around me in my search of professional fulfillment and financial well-being.

Note to the Reader

At the start of the book, I shared a traumatic event when I was a boy—a manic episode with my mom. You may be curious or concerned to know how she's doing. Mental illness is not an easy road to travel, and I'd like to share what an amazing and positive life my mom has made for herself and our family.

By taking control of the triggers of healthy, mental living, she has managed her condition religiously; adhering to her medication regime along with timely monitoring by her physicians and routine discussions with her therapists. She is surrounded by an environment of love and support from my brother and I and our close family. Most important is my dad, who has been by her side through it all. He's been a role model for me, not only in my relationship with my family, but by showing me what it means to be an honest, committed, and supportive man.

Another critical element allowing my mom to maintain her health and well-being is her strong faith and time spent actively involved with the community in all the places we've lived. Perhaps all is best summed up through her loving devotion to our family and especially her grandson Jack. My Mom's experience living a balanced, harmonious, and full life has been a vital example for me to draw upon as I face my own condition and land on my feet.

It has been over four years since I altered my professional path to live in greater harmony with my health and well-being. You may be curious to know how it's going.

I still see MS as my greatest teacher. To view things any other way would be counter to my healing interests. I have learned Multiple Sclerosis is a term the medical community uses to explain a phenomenon that they have no idea why occurs. Though I've found no root cause or cure, I continue to investigate the source of my symptoms.

If you were to pass me on the street you might not notice the imbalance when I walk; my right side—considerably stronger and neurologically more responsive than my left; you probably wouldn't see the atrophy in my left calf and hamstring, the loss of feeling in my finger tips, and you wouldn't feel the chronic stiffness in my neck, right shoulder and hips, the arthritis in my right knee, and the fatigue deep in my bones that I just can't shake. I have no complaints though; this is just the way it is for me.

I try to get half of my daily caloric intake from unprocessed raw food to minimize the energy my body requires to metabolize food. I maintain a vegan diet, minimize my sugar intake, drink only water, green tea, and an occasional glass of red wine, and I avoid casein and gluten—dairy and wheat proteins, though I occasionally fall off the wagon here. I've deviated from the strict detox and body cleansing diet because the lifestyle became too constricting, took too much time, and strained my relationship with Robyn.

I workout with a personal trainer twice a week, try and attend yoga class twice a week, walk one to three miles each day, and meditate regularly. I meet with my neurologist two to three times per year, inject myself with Copaxone, one of the half dozen MS drug therapies, every night, and inject myself with a $22,000 steroid a few times per year.

My "clean," regimented lifestyle allows me to write, play baseball with Jack and live in harmony with Robyn. Because my symptoms persist, I continue to look for why my body is attacking itself. Based on my lifestyle, I should be a vibrant vision of health, but I'm not. The re-appearance of symptoms, after what I experienced at OHI, leads me to believe that I might be putting something into my body that is causing the damage.

Perhaps there is an auto-immune response to something I'm eating (like the occasional wheat or dairy I consume when I fall of the wagon) that is leading to myelin destruction. I also wonder if the protein is not being introduced into my body, but rather is something my body makes on its own. However it gets there, I'm curious if a rogue protein might be attacking my myelin. An auto-immune response, after all, is at the heart of what is known about multiple sclerosis.

In a recent study of 397 people with MS, researchers from the University of California, San Francisco have identified that 47% have a protein, KIR4.1, not found in any of the 59 people in the control group of people without the disease. Maybe science has found the culprit. I have no idea whether this scenario is what's happening to me, but it gives me hope.

Maybe the demyelization has nothing to do with what I put into my body, but rather is due to some deep rooted structural issue. Maybe my body suffers the effects of chronic cerebro-spinal venus insufficiency (CCSVI), *a condition where people have obstructed blood flow in the veins that drain the central nervous system (the brain and spinal cord). Research indicates that CCSVI is significantly correlated with multiple sclerosis.*[1, 2,3,4] *As a result of these venous abnormalities, the blood flow rate through the central nervous system back toward the heart may become slowed, and blood may reflux back toward the brain and spine.*[1]

This is the condition that the Italian vascular surgeon, Dr. Paolo Zamboni, discovered and treated over ten years ago to relieve the MS symptoms his wife was experiencing. Groundbreaking research is being done today in the United States and Canada to better understand the condition. CCSVI may turn out to be a red herring in the treatment of MS. Studies show inconsistent and inconclusive results. Some support a link between CCSVI and MS while others don't. Regardless of the correlation between MS and CCSVI, more inquiry is required to understand conclusively whether CCSVI leads to MS, and if so to identify safe, effective, and repeatable courses for treatment.

Maybe the demyelization is due to some other deep rooted structural issue in my body like the presence of the two dead root canalled teeth in my jaw. You might recall the decision I made five years earlier to repair the cracked root canal and heal the infection above my front, root canalled tooth. I chose not to extract both teeth at the time. However, because my symptoms have persisted, I read up on the health impacts of root canalled teeth and am considering pursuing this surgery.

I found some interesting insights in the book the *Root Canal Cover-Up* by Dr. George Meinig, a distinguished endodonist and past president of the American Association of Endodonists, about root canalled teeth and chronic disease. The book uncovers the forgotten findings of Dr. Weston Price, who had studied the effects of root canalled teeth on rabbits. Dr Price found that rabbits with root canalled teeth sown under their skin suffered MS-like neurological symptoms that caused them to lose use of their back legs and die within two weeks.

Dr. Prince theorized that microscopic tubules in the teeth, known as dentin, harbored bacteria that leaked out of the teeth and metastasized throughout the body. His research was discredited by the formal medical community at the time *not* because of his research techniques, but because of how he used the theory of metastasis to explain the spread of bacteria throughout the body. The concept of metastasis is commonly accepted today. It explains how cancer spreads throughout the body.

I now wonder if the bacteria, that was once in my teeth, spread to my neck and other parts of my body causing the arthritis and related stiffness and pain. The medical community is suspiciously silent about Dr. Price's theory about the impact of root canalled teeth on health. When I made the decision to proceed with the less extreme procedure to deal with the infection in my mouth, I did so hoping that somehow fixing the cracked root canalled tooth and healing the infected soft tissue would improve my health. Now, I wonder if I should have completely removed the dead teeth to clear up the remaining symptoms. I have nothing to lose other than what's left of my teeth, time for the procedure and healing, and a few thousand dollars. I still have aspirations of running a 10K, and this procedure might hold the key.

Despite my symptoms, I remain optimistic. I've found my way back to setting goals and following through on the work to achieve them. But there's an important difference between how I approach life today compared to the days of my ego driven, health compromising perspective. I've found a way to set goals and live a healthy, productive, and harmonious existence in alignment with myself, my family, and those around me. I'm hopeful about potential breakthroughs that will lead to the end of my symptoms, but I don't let them define what I can or cannot do.

I'm a husband, a father, a son, a brother, a friend, and a writer. I live the healthiest and most vibrant life I can and want to assist others to find their best life, too. I carry the message that one path to achieving your goals is to listen to your body; remain open to ways of thinking, being, and acting in support of your life vision; surround yourself with an affirming support system, and make the necessary lifestyle changes to support the life you want.

I have a blog where I share more about my philosophy for VIBRANT living and am available as a coach and speaker. If you'd like to connect or work together, please visit my website at jonchandonnet.com or contact me at jon@vibrantlivingpress.com.

Acknowledgements

I am fortunate to be surrounded by so many whose love, support, encouragement and insights have contributed to the creation and shaping of this book. To my wife—my life partner; your love rounds out my experience; your presence soothes my troubles; your tough questions challenge me and allow me to see things that make me a better person; your strength is infectious. To my Mom and Dad—I appreciate every thing you've done to make this a reality. You provided a nurturing environment that allowed me to soar into adulthood, but it was when I crashed that you provided the most support and showed me what it means to love unconditionally and have faith in the unknown. To my brother—you've always been by my side whether at the finish line of a marathon or as the inspiration for my turn around, I couldn't have done this without you.

To the team of people who worked with me on a daily basis over the past eight years to help me chart the course from a source of inspiration to a finished product.

Holly Payne and the team at Skywriter Books—you had the faith and courage to take me on as a writing client and tirelessly worked with me. You nurtured, supported, and challenged me, then when I completed a draft, you and your editing team, worked with me to shape, mold, and polish my writing. Thank you! The words hardly capture how much gratitude I feel for all you have done.

Jonathan Fields and Jayme Johnson at Tribal Author—you helped me understand the path I needed to navigate to publish, you gave me context on how to build my platform, and you gave me the confidence to begin my journey.

Jayme Johnson, Matt Johnson, and the team at Worthy Marketing Group—you have worked with me daily over the last year to put the finishing touches on the book, helped me build my platform, strategized on how to best reach out to readers, and are doing the work to make connections.

The Moore family—your generosity allowed me to enlist the editorial services I needed.

Jack Barnard—you showed me how to go inside and connect to my truth when speaking and have shown me what it means to be a speaker.

I appreciate all you've done to support me. Thank you!

REFERENCES:

All references listed below pertain to content from the website CCSVI.org, a site for the CCSVI Alliance. They pertain to content referenced on the About page of that site retrieved September 24, 2013.

1. Zamboni P, Galeotti R, Menegatti E, et al. Chronic cerebrospinal venous insufficiency in patients with multiple sclerosis. Journal of Neurology, Neurosurgery, and Psychiatry. 2009; 80: 392-399

2. Al-Omari MH, Rousan, LA. Internal jugular vein morphology and hemodynamics in patients with multiple sclerosis. International Angiology. April, 2010; 29(2):115-120

3. Simka M, Kestecki J, Zaniewski M, Majewski E, Hartel M. Extracranial Doppler sonographic criteria of chronic cerebrospinal venous insufficiency in the patients with multiple sclerosis. International Angiology. April, 2010; 29(2): 109-114

4. Zivadinov, R. Preliminary Result

CPSIA information can be obtained at www.ICGtesting.com
Printed in the USA
LVOW10*1441220514

386940LV00010B/146/P

9 780615 836560